Live longer

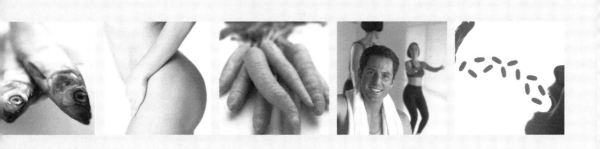

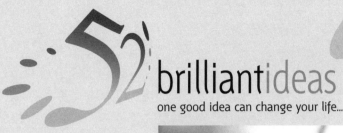

52 brilliantideas

one good idea can change your life...

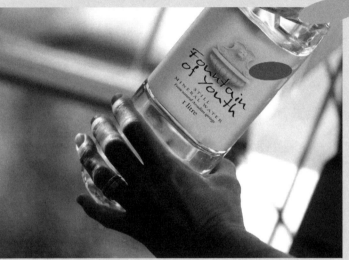

Live longer

Your whole health route to
longer life

Sally Brown

Careful now

We want your life to be long, rich, and rewarding but that doesn't mean we want to live it for you. You're a grown up now so it's up to you to take responsibility for your own life. Any alteration in the way you go about your life can affect its quality so you should consult your doctor or healthcare provider before changing your diet, undertaking any kind of change to your exercise routine or taking any nutritional supplements.

If you have any health problems of any nature – physical, emotional or mental – always consult the proper healthcare providers.

Although the contents of this book were checked at the time of going to press, the world keeps moving and the World Wide Web does so twice as fast. This means the publisher and author cannot guarantee the contents of any of the websites mentioned in the text.

Copyright © The Infinite Ideas Company Limited, 2005

The right of Sally Brown to be identified as the author of this book has been asserted in accordance with the Copyright, Designs and Patents Act 1988

First published in 2005 by
The Infinite Ideas Company Limited
36 St Giles
Oxford
OX1 3LD
United Kingdom
www.infideas.com

A CIP catalogue record for this book is available from the British Library.

ISBN 1-904902-27-8

Brand and product names are trademarks or registered trademarks of their respective owners.

Designed and typeset by Baseline Arts Ltd, Oxford
Printed and bound by TJ International, Cornwall

Brilliant ideas

Brilliant features

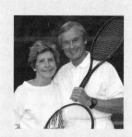

Each chapter of this book is designed to provide you with an inspirational idea that you can read quickly and put into practice straight away.

Throughout you'll find four features that will help you to get right to the heart of the idea:

■ *Here's an idea for you* Take it on board and give it a go – right here, right now. Get an idea of how well you're doing so far.

■ *Try another idea* If this idea looks like a life-changer then there's no time to lose. *Try another idea* will point you straight to a related tip to enhance and expand on the first.

■ *Defining idea* Words of wisdom from masters and mistresses of the art, plus some interesting hangers-on.

■ *How did it go?* If at first you do succeed, try to hide your amazement. If, on the other hand, you don't, then this is where you'll find a Q and A that highlights common problems and how to get over them.

Introduction

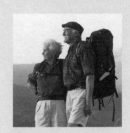

Remember when the best thing about being 60 was getting a free bus pass? Now, 60 is the new 40. We're surrounded by energetic sexagenarians who celebrate their sixtieth year by running across the Sahara, trekking to Kathmandu or signing up for a university degree. Yet as recently as 1930, you'd be lucky to even make it to your sixtieth birthday.

Most people can now expect to reach 80, but could we be living even longer? It certainly looks that way. According to some anti-ageing scientists, only 1 in 10,000 people actually die of old age – the vast majority die prematurely. Cell culture studies show that, biologically, our true lifespan could be 120 years. The world's longest-living woman, Jeanne Calment from France, died recently after reaching 122.

Of course, adding on an extra decade or two is pretty pointless if you spend them dozing in front of the TV in a nursing home. Living longer must go hand in hand with staving off disease, staying mentally sharp and simply having the energy to be enthusiastic about getting up in the morning.

It helps if you have a reason for staying younger for longer. For me, the idea really hit home when I had children at the fairly late age of 35. Suddenly, it became clear that I needed to put in some groundwork immediately if I wasn't to be a decrepit embarrassment of a mother by the time they reached their teens. And I also wanted to make sure I was still around when they had children – even if they left it as late as I had.

Once you start looking into the science of ageing, you realise it's big business. There's some fascinating research taking place – and some very questionable claims being made. As yet, there's no magic pill that stops ageing. In fact, over fifty top anti-ageing scientists recently signed a position statement to confirm this, railing against manufacturers cashing in by offering so-called 'wonder' supplements. But the experts agree that the way you live your life today has a big impact on how fit and well you'll be tomorrow and every single day after that. If your aim is to live longer, the best way to do it is achieve optimal health now and maintain it in the future.

No doubt you're now thinking of that one person you know who did all the wrong things and still managed to live to a ripe old age. I need look no further than my own grandfather who lived to 89, despite smoking a pack of cigarettes and downing several pints of beer a day. But look a little closer and you'll see that there's more going on than just genetic good luck. In almost all cases, there'll be some redeeming lifestyle factor that was strong enough to cancel out the negative health habits. In my granddad's case, it was probably that he was never overweight, walked miles every day, ate a simple diet of fresh local produce and didn't know the meaning of the word stress. And who knows how much longer he might have lived if he'd cut down on the beer and given up tobacco?

Giving your body the best chance of fighting off ageing means simply removing as many damaging elements as possible – smoking, stress, junk food – and boosting the things that research shows us protect our bodies – the right foods, exercise and social support. You'll find 52 ideas in this book for changing your lifestyle to promote a youthful life. I'm not expecting anyone to start at the beginning and make every single change. Some ideas will appeal, others won't. Some (giving up smoking, taking up exercise, losing weight) require more commitment and effort than others (flossing your teeth, taking a multivitamin, drinking tea). But make just one change a week – and stick with it – and gradually you should feel your energy levels rise and your overall sense of well-being improve. If you've picked this book off the shelf, the chances are that you already have an interest in living a healthy life. My aim with these ideas is to inspire you further and help you reach your full health potential. And even have some fun while you're doing it...

You may be asking yourself at this point if it will be worth the effort. The answer to that is yes – if you want the energy, strength and mobility for daily tasks, active hobbies and holidays, and if you want to be able to fight off illness and recover quickly from physical and psychological setbacks. Give your lifestyle an anti-ageing makeover now and you won't need to dread getting older. And you'll have a lot more to look forward to on your sixtieth birthday than a free bus pass!

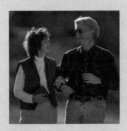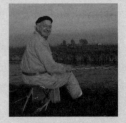

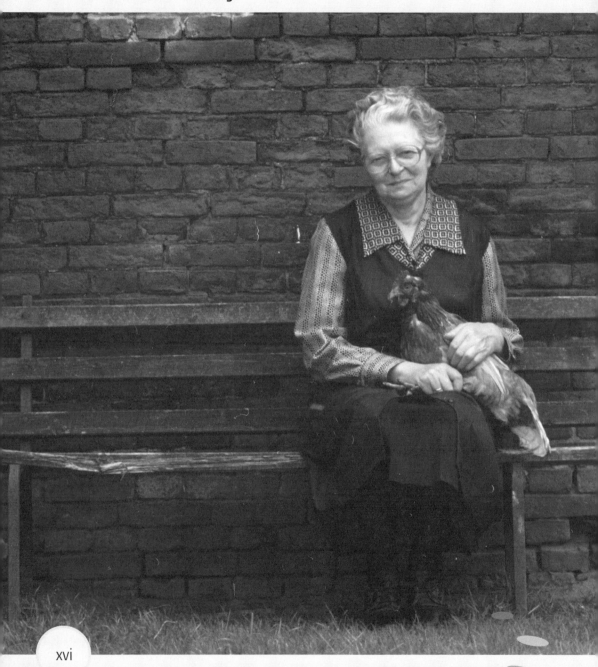

1

Ageing explained

We're undergoing a quiet revolution in our understanding of ageing. It may not be inevitable – and one day may even be reversible.

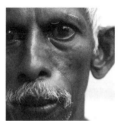

Slowing ageing down, right now, is something we can all do. It can be as easy as simply eating more vegetables.

What, exactly, is ageing all about? It's the subject of hot debate among scientists. Some see it as an unavoidable process that we can only slow down by postponing ageing-related diseases as long as possible. Others see it as a specific biological process that one day we may learn how to switch off.

For decades, it was thought that ageing was a way of getting rid of a generation of people who had already reproduced and so were no longer useful to the survival of the species. But in 1956 US scientist Dr Denham Harmon came up with the theory that ageing wasn't simply a sign that our time was nearly up – it was the result of the build-up of faults in the body. And these faults are caused by damage from unstable molecules called free radicals.

Here's an idea for you...

What's the simplest way to add more healthy years to your life? Drink more water. Drink more than five glasses a day and you'll halve your risk of certain cancers. But according to one recent survey, most of us drink fewer than four glasses of water every day. Why not buy a filter jug that fits in the fridge? Then you'll have cool, clean tasting water 'on tap'. Aim for two litres (around ten glasses) a day.

Free radicals are by-products of normal bodily processes – like breathing, eating and drinking – which are 'unstable' as they lack an electron, so they career around the body looking for spare electrons to bind with. In optimal health, the body simply mops up free radicals and makes them harmless. But if the body's self-repair capabilities weaken, free radicals, and the damage they cause, can accumulate, leading to serious diseases, muscle and bone wastage, reduced skin elasticity, weakened sight and hearing and slower mental reactions. Everything we associate with getting old. But this can be slowed down by eating more vegetables – they contain antioxidants which bind with free radicals and make them harmless.

One of the newest theories is called the cross-linking theory of age or the glycosylation theory of ageing. It's all about how glucose (sugar) binds to protein, causing damage. It's thought that a lot of skin-ageing and heart problems may be due to cross-linking. One theory is that sugars binding to DNA may cause damage that leads to malformed cells and thus to cancer. Excessive cross-linking is thought to be the reason why people with diabetes (who often have excess amounts of glucose in the body) tend to age quicker. So simply cutting back on the sugar in your diet may help keep you younger for longer.

Defining idea...

'The old believe everything; the middle aged suspect everything; the young know everything.'
Oscar Wilde

2

Recently, we've learned more about the role our DNA plays in the ageing process. Our DNA is our individual blueprint, passed to us from our parents. It means that we are born with a unique code and a predetermined tendency to certain types of physical and mental functioning that regulate the rate at which we age.

Free radicals aren't escaping political prisoners – they're your biggest enemy in the war against ageing. Read more on how to keep them at bay in IDEA 5, *Fighting free radicals.*

Try another idea...

These days, not a week goes by without a 'gene' headline hitting the papers: 'Researchers find the breast cancer gene', 'Colon cancer gene isolated'. This has given all the fatalists among us a new excuse for avoiding healthy lifestyle choices by saying, 'What's the point? It's all in the genes anyway.' It's the current equivalent of 'you could get run over by a bus tomorrow'. Yes, scientists have discovered that genetic mutations occurring in what are known as our 'germ line' cells, those that become the egg and sperm, can be passed from parent to child, creating a higher risk of developing certain diseases. And it's undoubtedly true that our deepening understanding of DNA will have far-reaching effects on our health in the future. But it's also important to keep it in perspective. The vast majority of diseases are caused by environmental (i.e. lifestyle) factors rather than genes. In breast cancer, for example, genetic predisposition is thought to account for less than 4% of cases. Inheriting a gene that increases your risk of developing a certain disease does *not* mean you're destined to get it.

'Just as we can alter the lifespan of a car by how well or badly we drive and maintain it, we alter the ageing of our body by how well, or badly, we take care of it.'
Top UK longevity expert Dr Tom Kirkwood

Defining idea...

Defining idea...

'Old age is the most
unexpected of all the things
that can happen to a man.'
Leon Trotsky

Scientists all over the world are studying these and many other theories in the hope that one day, we'll find a foolproof way to stop the ageing process. But until that day there is much you can do to influence the rate at which you age – simply by adapting the way you live your life.

How did it go?

Q   I feel a bit overwhelmed by all the changes I'm going to have to make to my life. Can you help?

A   *I'm not denying that there are plenty of suggestions for living a younger, longer life, but I'm not suggesting you do all of them at once. Making just one or two changes at a time will be your first step towards the optimal, healthy lifestyle you need in order to live younger for longer.*

Q   What's the optimum age to start fighting the ageing process? I'm 60 – have I left it too late?

A   *It's never too late! Lifestyle changes made now can help slow your rate of ageing immediately. Stop smoking, for instance, and your risk of a heart attack falls to half that of a smoker within a year. And 90-year-olds who start weight-training have been shown to gain muscle strength. So don't waste another day.*

2

Are you younger than you think?

Take this quiz and find out your true biological age.

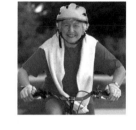

Ever told a tiny white lie and knocked off a few years when someone asks you how old you are? You may be being more honest than you think.

Scientists believe that as well as a calendar age, you also have a biological or 'body' age, which is determined by your health and lifestyle. We all know people who seem younger than their years – and those who seem old before their time. Now scientists believe that it's possible to have a biological age or body age of 50 in our seventies. We're only just realising that how fast, or how slowly, we age is a process that's under our control. We now know that our diet, activity levels, and even our emotional health all have a direct effect on the ageing process. How long your body and mind stay fit, active and healthy is determined by how you live your life.

Here's an idea for you... **The static balance test is an instant way of assessing your biological age. Stand barefoot on a flat surface with your feet together and your eyes closed. Raise your right foot six inches off the ground (if you're left-handed, raise your left foot). See how many seconds you can maintain your balance without having to open your eyes or put your foot down. Here are the approximate values (time in seconds before falling over) for different biological ages.**

- **04 seconds – 70 years**
- **05 seconds – 65 years**
- **07 seconds – 60 years**
- **08 seconds – 55 years**
- **09 seconds – 50 years**
- **12 seconds – 45 years**
- **16 seconds – 40 years**

It's only a matter of time before scientists devise a definitive method of determining true body age. And who knows, in the future, perhaps we'll come to discard birth dates altogether and use personal age assessments instead for employers, insurers – maybe even dating agencies!

In the meantime, try the quiz below to find out how you're ageing so far. Don't be dismayed if it's not good news. There's plenty of information to help you knock years off your true age and keep your biological age as young as possible.

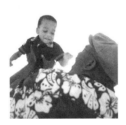
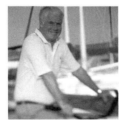
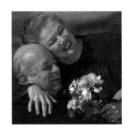

WHAT'S YOUR BODY AGE?

Start with your calendar age. If you can answer 'yes' to any of the following questions, add or subtract years as directed to find your body age.

See what changes you can make in just one day to add years to your life at IDEA 3, *What a difference a day makes...*

Try another idea...

1. Do you get at least thirty minutes of moderate exercise (like walking) on most days?
   YES – subtract 1 year

2. Do you exercise really intensively on a regular basis?
   YES – add 3 years

3. Do you rarely, if ever, do any physical exercise?
   YES – add 2 years

4. Are you more than 10% over the recommended weight for your height?
   YES – add 3 years

5. Are you the correct weight for your height?
   YES – subtract 1 year

6. Are you under stress or pressure on a regular basis?
   YES – add 4 years

7. Do you actively practise stress-reducing techniques such as meditation or yoga?
   YES – subtract 3 years

8. Have you experienced three or more stressful life events in the past year (for example divorce, bereavement, job loss, moving house)?
   YES – add 3 years

9. Do you smoke?
   YES – add 6 years

10. Do you have a cholesterol level of 6.7 or higher?
    YES – add 2 years

11. Do you have blood pressure that's 135/95 or over?
    YES – add 3 years

12. Do you eat five or more portions of a range of fresh fruit and vegetables every day?
    YES – subtract 5 years

13. Do you regularly eat processed, packaged or fast food?
    YES – add 4 years

14. Are you a vegetarian?
    YES – subtract 2 years

15. Do you eat oily fish three times a week?
    YES – subtract 2 years

16. Do you drink two or three small glasses of red wine, up to five days a week?
    YES – subtract 3 years

17. Do you drink more than 21 units of alcohol a week (if you're a man) or 14 (if you're a woman)?
    YES – add 5 years

18. Do you have an active social life and a supportive network of friends and family?
    YES – subtract 2 years

19. Do you have an active sex life?
    YES – subtract 2 years

20. Are you happily married?
    YES – subtract 1.5 years.

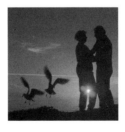

'*I was wise enough to never grow up while fooling most people into believing I had.*'
Margaret Mead, anthropologist

Defining idea...

How did it go?

Q **I'm a bit worried – I'm five years older than I thought I was. What should I do?**

A *Don't worry. Lowering your biological age is easier than you think – all it takes is some simple lifestyle changes. And I mean simple: could you handle drinking more tea, flossing your teeth and learning a new hobby? They'll all make you biologically younger. OK, there are some changes that require more effort, such as changing your diet, losing weight and exercising more, but you don't have to make every change at once. Take one step at a time and you'll soon see results.*

Q **Great – I'm much younger than my calendar age. Can I take it easy then?**

A *Well done! You're obviously already doing lots of the right stuff – eating plenty of fresh fruit and veg, getting some moderate exercise and avoiding stress. But don't rest on your laurels; now's the time to consolidate all your good work and ensure you have years of health and vitality ahead.*

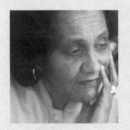 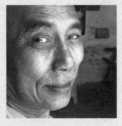

3

What a difference a day makes...

Motivated by instant results? These simple lifestyle changes could add years to your life in one day.

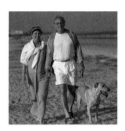

There are many different ways to stay younger for longer — eating different foods, cutting others out of your diet, exercising, getting out and about, watching your stress levels, taking the right vitamins.

It can seem overwhelming, but in practice it comes down to common sense. Most of it is even fun! To give you a better idea, here's what an ideal anti-ageing day could look like.

7.30 a.m. ALWAYS START YOUR DAY WITH BREAKFAST. People who eat breakfast live longer than people who don't – as long as they choose wholegrain-based cereals. Add a cup of green tea and a piece of fruit to boost your levels of disease-fighting antioxidants.

Here's an idea for you...

Defining your anti-ageing goals will make them more achievable. Try conjuring up an image of yourself as you'd like to be in a year's time. Someone who enjoys exercising three times a week, cooks imaginative, healthy dishes and has a fulfilling social life? Someone who's 12 kg lighter, who's given up smoking and who sticks to 14 units (or 21 if you're a man) of alcohol a week? Write down weekly steps that will get you to your goal. This week, it could be buying a new recipe book and learning to cook with pulses. Next week, it could be joining a local running group.

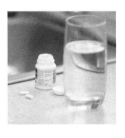

7.45 a.m. DRINK A GLASS OF WATER AND TAKE A MULTIVITAMIN. Most people don't get the recommended daily allowance of many essential vitamins and minerals. You're more likely to remember to take a supplement every day if you take it with breakfast.

8 a.m. BRUSH AND FLOSS YOUR TEETH – it can take six years off your biological age. The bacteria that cause gum disease also cause furring of the arteries which can lead to heart disease. And bad teeth never helped anyone look younger!

8.30 a.m. WALK TO WORK. Exercising for at least thirty minutes every day is the best way to keep your heart and lungs in good shape (not to mention the rest of you).

9 a.m. DRINK A GLASS OF WATER and try to have six more throughout the day.

10 a.m. HAVE ANOTHER CUP OF TEA. Always squeeze your teabag – you'll release twice as many antioxidants that way.

10.30 a.m. CONNECT WITH YOUR FRIENDS and colleagues by email or phone. People with a strong social network of friends and family live longer and healthier lives than more solitary types.

If you're tickled by the idea that laughing a lot helps you live longer, find out why at IDEA 29, *Game for a laugh*.

Try another idea...

12.30 p.m. DO SOME LUNCHTIME YOGA. It balances out all the body's systems and gets your organs working efficiently. Ever wondered why yoga teachers look so young?

1.30 p.m. HAVE A RAINBOW SALAD FOR LUNCH. Use as many differently coloured vegetables – red peppers, watercress, grated carrot and courgette, young spinach leaves, cherry tomatoes – as you can. Dress with olive oil and balsamic vinegar, and sprinkle with a handful of toasted sunflower and sesame seeds for the perfect antioxidant-packed, disease-fighting lunch.

3.30 p.m. TAKE THE STAIRS. Climb up and down a flight six times a day and you'll prevent weight gain of 2 kg a year. You take 36 days off your life for every 5 kg overweight you are.

6 p.m. MEDITATE ON THE TRAIN HOME. You'll lower your blood pressure and slow your heartbeat, both of which are good for your heart's health. Close your eyes and breathe

'The best thing about the future is that it comes only one day at a time.'
Abraham Lincoln

Defining idea...

deeply, in through your nose and out through your mouth. Try to empty your mind and simply concentrate on what the breath feels like as it enters your nostrils and leaves through your lips. Feel it filling your lungs and pushing out your abdomen. Keep this focus for around ten to fifteen minutes.

7 p.m. HAVE A SMALL GLASS OF RED WINE. Go for a deep red like a Pinot Noir for a maximum boost of disease-fighting flavonoids. Just be sure to stop at one or two.

8 p.m. HAVE SALMON FOR DINNER. Oily fish like salmon – or mackerel, sardines, trout or tuna – keeps your brain healthy and can stave off Alzheimer's if eaten at least twice a week.

9 p.m. WATCH A FUNNY VIDEO. Laughter boosts your immune system and reduces the ageing effect of stress hormones on the body. So switch off the news and watch a comedy instead.

10 p.m. HAVE SEX. People who have sex more than twice a week live longer than those who don't.

11 p.m. SLEEP! It's your body's chance to release growth hormone and repair itself from the inside out. So never skimp on your shut-eye – aim for at least six to eight hours a night.

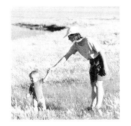
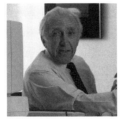
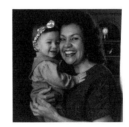

Q   **It's easy to stick to a healthy regime for one day. But how do I find
the motivation to do it in the long term?**

A   *Hmm, there's something about the word 'regime' that conjures up uniforms,
shouting and being told to do stuff you don't want to do. Living younger
for longer can be a lot more fun than that. It's really about maximising your
potential well-being now and in the future. Once you get started, remember
this: if you stick to the principles 80% of the time, it'll work, and with a
little margin left over for indulgences.*

Q   **How will I know when all this hard work starts working?**

A   *Well, first of all, stop thinking of it as hard work. You're simply making some
lifestyle adjustments, some of which you'll find easier than others.
Timewise, once you start basing most of your diet on wholegrains, fresh
fruit and vegetables, pulses, oily fish or lean meat, you should start seeing
a boost in energy levels within two weeks – especially if you remember to
drink lots of water too. Add exercise and you should be sleeping better and
feeling generally less stressed within around three weeks. After four weeks,
other people should start to notice. They may simply tell you you're looking
well but I bet it won't be long before someone also says you're looking
younger. Get ready to field off questions about facelifts.*

*How did
it go?*

15

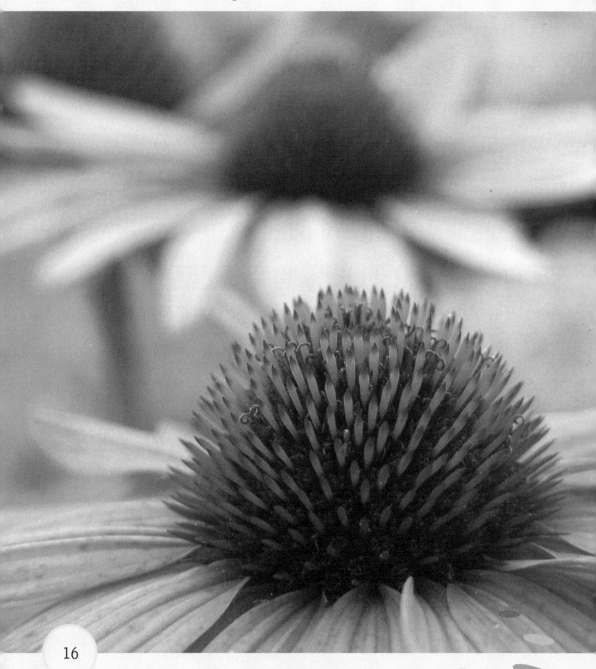

4

Boost your immune system

You can't live younger for longer without a strong immune system – it's your private army, fighting off invasion by foreign organisms that can lead to disease.

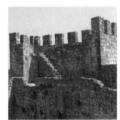

Here's how to keep your troops in peak condition and help prevent the illnesses we associate with ageing.

Every day, hordes of bugs (bacteria, viruses, parasites and fungi) are doing their best to get inside your body. To a bug, you're a very attractive proposition: a bijou residence offering warmth, safety and food.

Luckily the body has developed a highly effective defence system for keeping these bugs out. Inside you is an army of scavenging white blood cells, constantly roaming the body looking for invaders. If a scavenging cell spots one, then it's immediately transported to the nearest lymph glands (situated in the neck, armpits and groin) and destroyed before it's even had a chance to wave a white flag. (You can feel this brutal elimination process taking place when your lymph glands become swollen.)

Here's an idea for you...

Regular massage not only reduces stress and anxiety, it can also boost the immune system by increasing levels of infection-fighting cells. Can't coerce someone into doing it? Don't have the time or spare cash to see a professional? No problem – simply get a tennis ball, lean against a wall and roll the ball around between your back and shoulders and the wall. Try it – you'll be hooked.

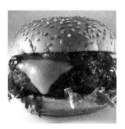

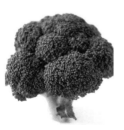

A healthy body with a fully functioning immune system sees off potentially dangerous organisms and carcinogens every day. It's even thought that cancer cells grow and are destroyed by the immune system on a regular basis. It's no surprise that a recent study of healthy centenarians found they had one thing in common: a healthy immune system.

The danger comes when the immune system is weakened, and invaders remain undetected and start to multiply. Some pathogens, such as HIV, are so powerful they simply trample over your body's defence system. But in most cases there are three main factors which lead to weak links in your inner defences: a less than ideal diet (an army marches on its stomach, after all), the environment in which you live (constantly challenging your defences over and above what's normal by smoking, sunbathing or breathing in toxic fumes), and mental well-being – feeling under stress on a regular basis.

YOU ARE WHAT YOU EAT

Your immune system works best when you keep it supplied with a full range of micronutrients such as vitamins and minerals. But even people who eat a balanced diet often show deficiencies and there are two theories about why. When we evolved, we were designed to lead active lives, hunting, gathering and escaping predators, and consuming 3000–4000 calories a day. Now we're mainly sedentary, and need around 2000 calories, we may not be able to eat enough to get the full range of micronutrients we need. The second theory is that today's intensive farming methods have depleted our soil of key minerals (such as selenium) and our food processing methods further deplete food of micronutrients. We now know that a large number of people are regularly missing out on vitamins A, D and B12; folic acid, riboflavin, iron, magnesium, zinc, copper and omega-3 oils. Plus, nutritionists think we're more likely to have deficiencies as we get older, because the digestive system becomes less efficient at absorbing micronutrients from the food we eat.

So strengthening your immune system starts with taking a good multivitamin and mineral supplement every day. By the way, simply buying the bottle and leaving it in the kitchen drawer doesn't work! You need to top up your micronutrients every day (so a bottle just lasts as long as it says on the label – 30, 60 or 90 days. Not all year). This really helps: there was a US study of older people with weakened immune systems. After taking a daily nutritional supplement they had fully functioning immune systems within a year.

There's truth in the saying that laughter is the best medicine. Find out how it boosts your immune system at IDEA 29, *Game for a laugh.*

Try another idea...

19

Defining
idea...

BE AWARE OF YOUR ENVIRONMENT

Your body has a regular army designed to fight off everyday invaders, and it also has a troop of 'special forces', called T-cells, held in reserve for extraordinary circumstances. But if you bombard your body with extra invaders on a regular basis, the effectiveness of these special forces is inevitably weakened, allowing disease-causing bugs to multiply. And while you can't control the many bacteria and viruses that assault your immune system every day, you do have control over additional toxic invaders such as cigarette smoke (whether first-hand or passive) and, to a lesser extent, environmental pollution.

THE MIND/BODY FACTOR

Undergoing stress on a regular basis is like offering a personal invitation to foreign invaders to walk through the chinks it causes in your defences. Many of the hormones involved in your body's fight or flight response – how it responds to stress – are actually immune suppressants, slowing down its natural disease-fighting mechanisms. Ever noticed how you're more prone to colds when you feel under pressure? It's not just your imagination. People in one study were most likely to develop a cold if they had experienced a negative life event in the past year. It's also been found that the effectiveness of a pneumonia vaccine was reduced if recipients were suffering from stress.

Q   I cycle to work along a fairly busy route – would driving be better for my immune system?

How did it go?

A   *No; in fact, the opposite is true. The pollution hotspot is in the centre of the road where cars drive. Pollution levels fall dramatically towards the side of the road where cyclists and pedestrians travel. So keep up the cycling!*

Q   What is the easiest way to tell if my immune system needs a boost?

A   *A good indication is how you shake off minor illnesses. Do you get more than two colds a year? Are cuts and grazes slow to heal? If so, you should start supporting your immune system today.*

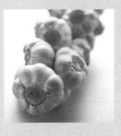 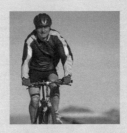 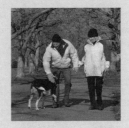

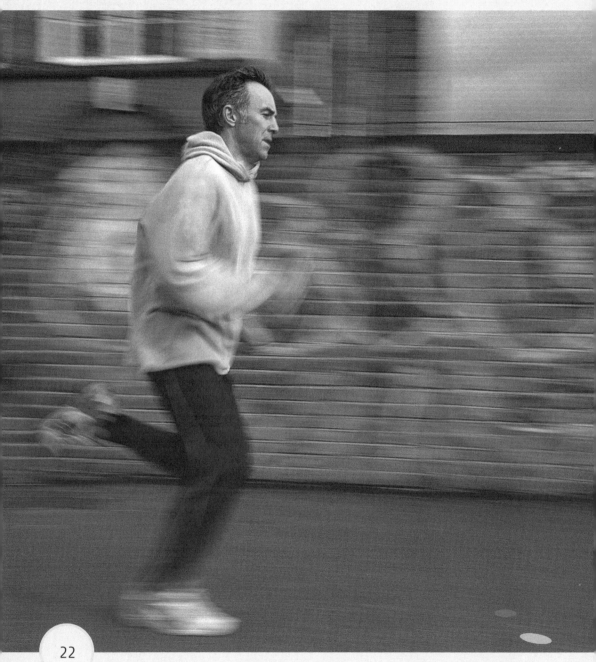

5

Fighting free radicals

You don't need to get radical to stave off ageing – you just need to help your body do its housework.

Ageing is not a straightforward process. One of its biggest paradoxes is that the very element that gives us life — oxygen — is also the thing that ages us most. But it can be combated.

When you put petrol in your car, you create energy – and noxious exhaust fumes. It's a similar story in the body. When you breathe, oxygen enters the bloodstream and combines with fats and carbohydrates to create the energy that every cell in your body needs in order to function. But a by-product is created during the process – an unstable molecule called a free radical or oxidant. This roams the body, bombarding your body's cells, trying to steal electrons to make itself 'stable'.

According to one estimate, free radicals attack each cell up to 10,000 times a day. If they successfully attack the DNA, stored in the cell's nucleus, they can cause cancer. If they successfully attack the mitochondria, or the energy factories of the cell, they can stop them working efficiently. And, as the mitochondria supply energy for all the bodily organs and systems, the knock-on effect is felt as ageing in the body.

Here's a simple way to see the free radical effect working. Take an apple, cut it in half. Rub one half in lemon juice and leave both halves out for a couple of hours. When you come back, you'll have one brown half and one that's stayed white. The browning is the oxidation process at work. But rubbing cut fruits with lemon juice (which contains high levels of vitamin C, an antioxidant) delays the browning process. Now imagine what that vitamin C could do inside your body.

It's only been in the last two decades that we've really begun to understand the role that free radicals play in the ageing process. Free radical damage is thought to be the main cause of Alzheimer's, cancer, heart disease and inflamed joints, as well as wrinkles and liver spots. In fact, the rate at which you age is directly related to how well your body deactivates these oxygen radicals. It might explain why pigeons live 35 years, twelve times as long as rats, animals that are about the same size: for the amount of oxygen they take in, pigeons produce only half as many free radicals as rats. Some experts believe that if you can boost your defences against free radicals, you can extend your life.

Luckily, most free radicals are neutralised by an army of good guys in the body known as antioxidants. It's like a house always getting dirty, and the antioxidants always tidying it up. The best way to stave off ageing is to help your body keep on top of its housework. Here's how.

KEEP YOUR DEFENCES UP BY BOOSTING YOUR ANTIOXIDANTS

The easiest way to do this? Eat more fruit and veg! They're packed with antioxidants – which is why nutritionists are always banging on about getting your 'five a day'. Try to choose differently coloured fruit and vegetables every day and eat local and seasonal produce. The sooner fruits and vegetables are eaten after picking, the more nutrients they contain (imported produce can take anything from a month to a year to arrive in the UK after picking). Home-grown is best but visiting your nearest farmers' market or having an organic box delivered are great choices too. Check labels for origin in your supermarket and buy food produced locally.

Cutting back on calories can cut the number of free radicals formed. See IDEA 17, Less cake, more birthdays?

Try another idea...

DON'T ADD TO THE FREE RADICAL LOAD

That means giving up smoking, which loads the body with millions of free radicals every time you inhale. The free radicals in cigarettes cause the fat in your blood to oxidise and form plaques on the artery walls, which is why smokers have a raised risk of heart disease.

DON'T SUNBATHE

Exposure to ultraviolet light floods the skin with free radicals and causes 80–90% of skin ageing.

'Life is better than death, I believe, if only because it is less boring and because it has fresh peaches in it.'
Alice Walker, writer

Defining idea...

EXERCISE REGULARLY

Keep it moderate, though – great news for anyone who hates painful, red-in-the-face, exercise sessions. Intense exercise uses up large amounts of oxygen and produces large amounts of free radicals as a by-product. The body can't mop up the free radicals quick enough and damage can occur, which is why athletes can suffer from depressed immune systems. But this isn't carte blanche to become part of the sofa – *moderate* exercise stimulates the production of the body's antioxidant enzymes and slows the ageing process. Aim for a minimum of around thirty minutes of brisk walking a day.

Q **If free radical damage is caused by oxygen, would I live longer if I took shallower breaths?**

A *It's true that the faster you breathe, the more oxygen you take in and the more free radicals are formed in the body. This is why many athletes who exercise intensively often have depressed immune systems. But trying to restrict the breathing process is not the answer either, as without oxygen the cells in your body can't burn the food you eat and convert it into ATP, the energy molecule essential for growth and repair. What's important is ensuring your body has enough antioxidants to neutralise the free radicals being produced.*

Q **These free radicals sound scary. Can I really fight them with just fruit and veg?**

A *Antioxidants are your first line of defence against free radical damage, and the more fruit and veg in your diet, the more antioxidants you take in. It's why vegetarians live longer than meat-eaters. It's no coincidence, either, that the world's longest living people eat diets that are packed with fresh vegetables and fruit. The Okinawans in Japan, for instance, who boast more people over the age of 105 than anywhere else on the planet, eat between seven and ten daily servings of fruit and vegetables. So get chomping!*

6

Upping the anti

Antioxidants could add years to your life by fighting free radical damage – if you're getting enough.

You have an army of good guys — antioxidants — which roam the body, eliminating the free radicals they find. You can boost their ranks simply by eating the right foods.

It's always important to know your enemy and in the war against ageing, it's free radicals, the unstable molecules that are a by-product of breathing and which damage the body's cells. There's nothing you can do to stop free radicals forming (except stop breathing, which would be a bit, well, radical), but antioxidants can eliminate them.

One half of the antioxidant army consists of compounds and enzymes that the body makes itself, using micronutrients found in the diet such as selenium, zinc, manganese, copper, iron, lipoic acid and glutathione. The other half are antioxidants delivered in the food we eat including vitamins A, C, E and B, and the vitamin-like compounds flavonoids, carotenoids and coenzyme Q10.

Here's an idea for you...

Black really is beautiful when it comes to staving off ageing. The darker the pigment – think plums, prunes, bilberries, blackberries, dates and raisins – the higher the ORAC rating. It's thought the pigment is a rich source of antioxidants. To maximise the benefits, wash rather than peel the skin of fruits and veg – the pigment is often concentrated in the skin or outer leaves. Try to eat a dark red, purple or black fruit or vegetable every day. And if you love wine, go for deep reds – they contain the most flavonoids.

When you eat a diet high in antioxidants, a protective shield is created around each cell which fights off and destroys the attacking free radicals. But if you're depleted in any of these micronutrients, there will be cracks in the shield. Many scientists believe the rise in heart disease, Alzheimer's and some cancers can be directly linked to micronutrient depletion. Our intake of selenium, for example, has fallen by 50% in the past 50 years due to intensive farming methods that leach it from the soil.

When it comes to their antioxidant content, not all foods were created equal. Meat, fish and dairy products do contain antioxidants but they're destroyed by cooking. Fruit and vegetables, however, contain high levels of antioxidants that survive the cooking process (as long as you don't boil them to mush). For very basic good health, you need 'five a day' – five portions (a portion is around a handful) of fresh fruit and vegetables a day. But to fend off ageing you need to step up a level and pack in as many antioxidants as possible.

It's easier to do than you might think, thanks to the brilliant scientists at Tufts University in the States who have very helpfully rated the antioxidant value of every food. It's a system known as ORAC: oxygen radical absorption capacity. The higher the ORAC, the more powerful a food is at mopping up free radicals. In fact, eating plenty of high-ORAC foods could raise the antioxidant power of blood by 10–25%.

One Tufts study of 1300 older people showed that those who had two or more portions a day of dark-pigmented vegetables such as kale and spinach were only half as likely to suffer a heart attack – and had a third of the risk of dying of cancer – compared with people averaging less than one portion a day. Other research has shown that a diet of high-ORAC foods fed to animals prevents long-term memory loss and improves learning capabilities. It may be no coincidence that this high-ORAC diet is very similar to the one eaten by the Hunza people of the Indian Himalayas, who commonly live beyond 100.

Visit your health-food store and you'll see you can buy antioxidants as a supplement. But the researchers at Tufts think it's the whole foodstuff and the way the hundreds of micronutrients within it (some of which they're yet to identify) react *together* that provides its powerful antioxidant punch. If you're the cautious type, take a belt-and-braces approach – aim for a high-ORAC diet and add a good antioxidant supplement just in case.

There's another group of food that research suggests may have a valuable role in countering ageing: oily fish. For more on this, see IDEA 11, *Get hooked on fish*.

Try another idea...

'The amount of antioxidants that you maintain in your body is directly proportional to how long you will live.'
Dr Richard Cutler, anti-ageing researcher

Defining idea...

29

THE TOP ORAC-SCORING FOODS

The following figures are the number of ORACs that 100 grams of each food provides. A high-ORAC diet will provide 3000–5000 units a day.

Prunes, 5770

Raisins, 2830

Blueberries, 2400

Blackberries, 2036

Garlic, 1939

Kale, 1770

Cranberries, 1750

Strawberries, 1540

Spinach, 1260

Raspberries, 1220

Brussels sprouts, 980

Plums, 949

Alfalfa sprouts, 930

Broccoli, 890

Beetroot, 840

Avocado, 782

Oranges, 750

Red grapes, 739

Red peppers, 710

Cherries, 670

Kiwi fruit, 602

Baked beans, 503

Pink grapefruit, 483

Kidney beans, 460

Onion, 450

White grapes, 446

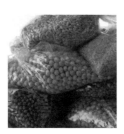 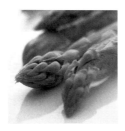 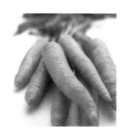

Q   **I'm not sure about this – isn't it really complicated?**

A   *Try thinking of it as simply adding to your diet rather than completely changing it. Try a handful of prunes or blueberries on your breakfast cereal in the morning. Stuff some spinach leaves or avocado into your chicken roll for lunch. Add a side dish of steamed red cabbage and raisins with your main meal, and munch on a plum or some red grapes when you have a break.*

Q   **I only really like a few vegetables (potatoes, carrots and broccoli) but I do eat a lot of them. Am I getting enough ORACs?**

A   *It's a start. The bad news is that potatoes contain limited numbers of antioxidants so they aren't counted in your 'five a day'. You really need to widen your repertoire because different vegetables and fruits contain different micronutrients which all have a role to play. Antioxidant compounds are responsible for the bright colours of fruit and vegetables – from yellows, oranges and reds to purples, blues and greens. Your best anti-ageing insurance policy is really to try to eat a rainbow of colours every day to get the widest range of antioxidants. Why not be adventurous and buy something you've never tasted before? If you always eat broccoli, try spring greens instead. Swap sweet potatoes for ordinary potatoes, or add celeriac to your mash. Have you ever started the day with a berry smoothie or a fresh fig?*

How did
it go?

31

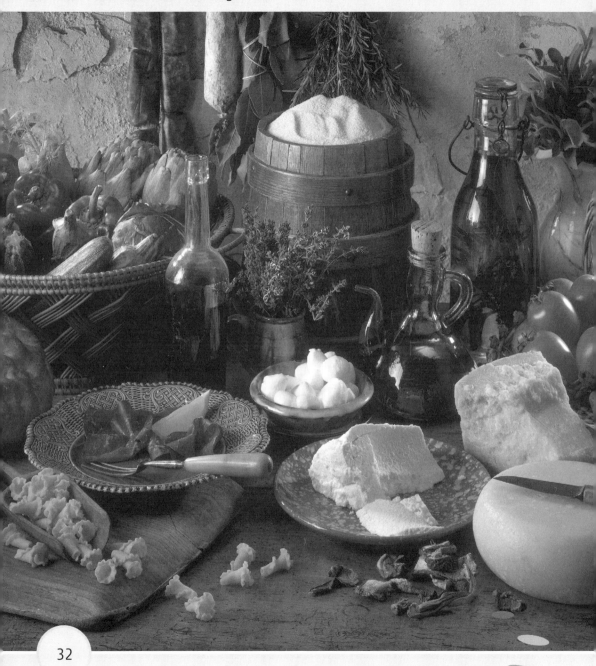

7

Your anti-ageing diet

**Every meal you eat is an opportunity to fend off ageing, so
eat the right foods.**

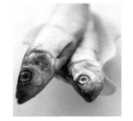

If feeling and looking younger than your
years is important to you, you'll have
already made the connection between your
health and your fridge.

There's a good chance there'll be broccoli, spinach and carrots in there. You won't
have to rely on the lettuce in your burger for one of your five-a-day portions of fruit
and veg. You probably know from experience that some foods give you energy and
make you feel full of vitality, and others drag you down. You're well on the road to
the perfect anti-ageing diet. Now it's time for an upgrade.

Food is our most important weapon in the war against ageing and disease. You only
need to look at the differences in life expectancy around the world for proof. It's
why those Japanese living in Japan, eating a diet rich in fish, vegetables and soy, and
low in fat and sugar, have the longest lifespan and the lowest levels of heart disease.
It's also why women in Scotland are nine times more likely to die from a heart
attack than women in France.

Here's an idea for you...

Grow your own superfood at home – you don't even need a garden! Sprouts are young green plants germinated from the seeds of vegetables, nuts, grains or beans and they've got antioxidants in super-concentrated amounts. You can buy sprouting kits or just use a large jar and some clean muslin. Simply soak the seeds overnight, place in your sprouter, then rinse with water twice a day. Keep in a dark warm place and they should be ready to eat within three days – give them a boost of sunlight before eating, then just grab a handful to add fresh crunch to salads or sandwiches.

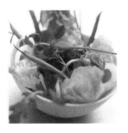

A disease-fighting, anti-ageing diet means cooking from scratch, buying fresh ingredients and including as many foods as possible that have been identified as 'superfoods'. Here are just a few of the easiest to find and cook with. Try introducing one or two a month and experimenting with ways to eat them.

SPINACH

It's all in the colour – spinach and other dark green vegetables such as kale, watercress, rocket and spring greens are packed with hundreds of disease-fighting micronutrients. Spinach is good at protecting eyesight as well as keeping the arteries clear of cholesterol, reducing blood pressure and lowering the risk of almost every type of cancer. Try using baby spinach leaves as a base for salads (it contains 90% more antioxidants than iceberg lettuce), adding them to stir-fries (right at the end – it barely needs cooking), or steaming them and serving as a side dish sprinkled with fresh lemon juice.

BROCCOLI

Broccoli is cancer's worst enemy. It comes from a family of cruciferous vegetables (including cabbage, kale and Brussels sprouts) that contain high levels of sulphur compounds which increase the enzymes that stop cancer cells growing. They also contain high levels of the antioxidant vitamin C and cholesterol-lowering fibre. If there are any leaves left on the stalk, don't discard them before cooking – they contain more carotenoids than the florets! Simply steam and serve, making a perfect accompaniment to meals.

As well as adding foods, you need to cut out those that will increase your risk of disease and speed up the ageing process. For more on this, see IDEA 16, Foods to lose.

Try another idea...

ONIONS

Onions are high in the flavonoid quercitin, which can cut heart disease risk by 755%. Flavonoids also boost the immune system. One study showed a strong link between regular consumption of onions and a reduced risk of stomach cancer.

SWEET POTATOES

While white potatoes provide low amounts of antioxidants, the orange-skinned sweet potato is packed with anti-cancer antioxidants. They can be baked in their skins, or boiled and mashed – or try cutting them into chunks and roasting them in the oven in a little olive oil to make chips.

'Are you getting enough sweet potato?'
A popular greeting among Okinawans, one of the world's longest-lived people

Defining idea...

NUTS

Nuts got a bad reputation during the 1980s fat-free diet craze – we still think of them as a naughty treat. They are high in calories, but in moderation (a handful, a few times a week) they can reduce your risk of having a heart attack by up to 50%. They're packed full of monounsaturates, which lower 'bad' LDL cholesterol and raise 'good' HDL cholesterol. Go for them raw rather than salted or roasted. They're delicious simply chopped, or toasted in a dry frying pan, and added to salads or sprinkled on soups.

WHOLEGRAINS

White, refined carbohydrates such as white bread, rice and pasta – plus refined flour products such as cakes, pastries and biscuits – have little to offer an anti-ageing diet. Refined flour is stripped of its disease-fighting fibre and nutrients. But foods that come from the wholegrain, those that still contain the antioxidant-packed wheatgerm, will help to lower your risk of heart disease, hypertension and certain cancers. So if 'whole' isn't the first word in the list of ingredients, ditch it.

YOGURT

Live bio-yogurt is a good anti-ageing food as it's full of probiotics or 'good bacteria' essential for healthy digestion and boosting the immune system. Getting your digestive system working effectively means you'll also get the most out of the other anti-ageing foods you're eating.

Q **I've heard that a raw food diet provides the most antioxidants. Is there any truth in this?**

How did it go?

A *It's true that cooking reduces the nutrient content of food (with the exception of tomatoes – cooking makes lycopene, the anti-cancer compound found in this fruit, more readily available to the body). Some people choose to eat all or most of their vegetables and fruit uncooked and say it's the key to staving off disease and boosting energy levels. It's also a challenging diet to stick to (especially in winter). A less extreme version is to steam or lightly stir-fry vegetables instead of boiling them and eat a vegetable-packed side salad with lunch or dinner every day.*

Q **What's best for anti-ageing – three meals a day or grazing on lots of snack meals?**

A *Some anti-ageing experts are keen on grazing – they say that snacking throughout the day puts less stress on the body and promotes better digestion than eating three larger meals. If this style of eating suits you, try opting for six 'mini-meals' a day, making sure you get a full range of fruit and vegetables, nuts, pulses, wholegrains and fish.*

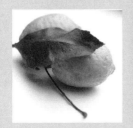 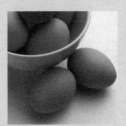 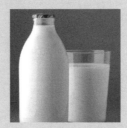

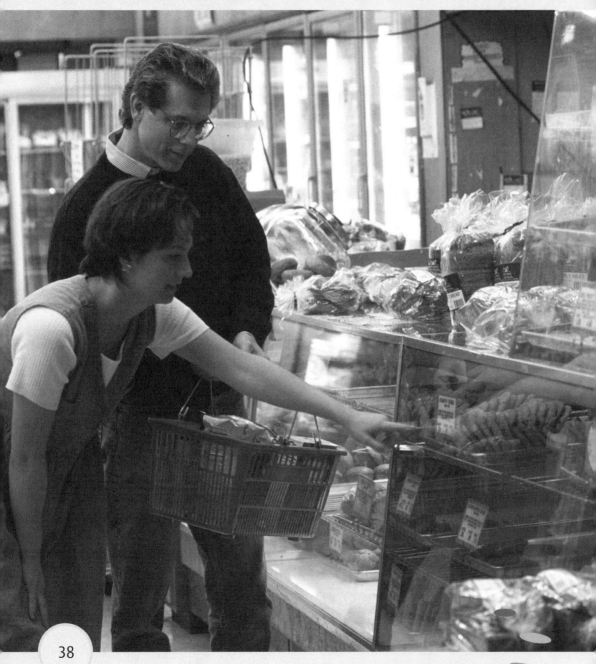

8

The anti-ageing store cupboard

It's time to go shopping. Supermarket shelves are full of anti-ageing superfoods – if you know what to look for.

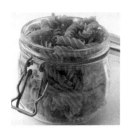

Not the most organised person on the planet? Prone to throwing together meals at the last minute from whatever's left in the fridge? You can still eat an anti-ageing diet.

Stock up your store cupboard with these everyday items that are all actually superfoods in disguise. Here are your shopping essentials.

TINNED SARDINES/HERRING/MACKEREL

A cheap, convenient and delicious way to get the all-important oily fish into the diet. No one should be without a stack of cans of sardines and similar oily fish, preferably in tomato sauce (a good source of cancer-fighting lycopene). If you're ever stuck for a simple supper idea, simply mash up a can with a squirt of lemon juice and serve on wholegrain toast. Delicious.

Here's an idea for you...

Don't forget to chew! Unchewed food is hard to digest and its micronutrients pass through our systems. The less you chew your superfoods, the less their micronutrients are absorbed. Aim to chew each mouthful fifteen times before swallowing.

TINNED TOMATOES

In the 1980s studies revealed that people who ate a lot of tomato-based foods were less likely to get prostate cancer. It's the lycopene, which gives the tomato the red colour, that makes it a superfood. What's more, this powerful antioxidant is most easily absorbed by the body when it's cooked – so tinned tomatoes (or tomato-based pasta sauces) are actually a better anti-ageing choice than fresh. Try them warmed and served on toast for breakfast.

TINNED BEANS

Beans or pulses are all full of polyphenols, an important antioxidant. Just eating beans four times a week could cut your risk of heart disease by 22%. They're also a great source of fibre which helps to reduce 'bad' cholesterol and raise 'good' cholesterol, and are good sources of potassium, calcium and magnesium which help to reduce hypertension. Soaking and cooking dried beans is more economical than using tins, but keeping tinned beans means you can easily add them to a salad, stew or soup. Which to choose? According to one study, the darker the bean, the higher the antioxidant levels, but they're all a good bet. Cooked, mashed kidney or black beans make a good tortilla filling – add a slice of avocado and a fresh tomato salsa for a nutritious taste boost. Or make home-made houmous – a tasty snack.

FROZEN VEGETABLES

Pack your freezer with frozen vegetables and there's no excuse for not eating them with every meal; they may even contain more nutrients than fresh vegetables that have been transported long distances. Most commercially produced frozen produce is frozen immediately after harvest when nutrient concentrations are at their highest. But bear in mind that the way you cook vegetables has a big effect on their nutrient content – lightly steamed is best. All vegetables boiled in large amounts of water for long periods of time lose far more of their nutritional content compared to vegetables that are lightly steamed.

FROZEN BERRIES

Berries, including bilberries, blackberries and cranberries, all contain high levels of anthocyanins – powerful antioxidants that work synergistically with vitamin C. Studies have shown that berries may slow or even reverse the ageing of the brain, preventing dementia. Keep a bag of frozen ones in the freezer and you can simply throw a handful into yogurt and blend for a ready-chilled smoothie. Frozen berries are also great added to hot porridge.

No store cupboard should be without a large bottle of olive oil. Find out why in IDEA 10, *Time for an oil change?*

Try another idea...

'It's clear that up to 70% of strokes and 80% of heart disease can be prevented by changes in diet and lifestyle.' Dr Balz Frei, director of the Linus Pauling Institute which researches the role of diet in disease

Defining idea...

DRIED FRUIT

Prunes, currants, cranberries and raisins all have a high ORAC rating – which means they're good at counteracting the damaging effects of free radicals in the body. Opt for organic varieties when you can (pesticides can be concentrated in dried fruits). Grab a handful as a snack, sprinkle them over a salad or add to your breakfast cereal in the morning.

PEANUT BUTTER

It's packed with healthy monounsaturates and may lower your heart disease risk by 21%. Go for a brand that has no added sugar or salt and no hydrogenated vegetable oils (trans fats). Try spreading it on wholegrain toast instead of margarine or butter or spread two tablespoons on half an apple for a satisfying snack.

CANNED PINEAPPLE

This is loaded with vitamin C, which can help maintain a strong immune system, and potassium, which protects your heart by regulating blood pressure. Add it to a stir-fry for sweet and sour flavour.

SOBA NOODLES

A Japanese staple, these noodles are made from buckwheat, a good source of two cancer-fighting antioxidants, quercetin and rutin. Use them in place of less nutritious egg noodles in stir-fries and soups.

Q   I've now got a fully stocked anti-ageing store cupboard. Trouble is, I eat out three times a week. What can I do?

How did it go?

A   *Simply think of what you'd eat at home and try to order as close to it as possible. Could you order a high-ORAC side dish such as steamed broccoli or spinach or a rocket salad? Is there a lycopene-packed, tomato-based pasta sauce on the menu? And if you're in a Chinese restaurant, could you order stir-fried vegetables with tofu or chicken and steamed rice?*

Q   What if I just can't cook?

A   *Well, it's never too late to learn – why not treat yourself to a healthy cookery course? Once you're a confident cook, you'll soon appreciate how relaxing and satisfying preparing meals from fresh ingredients can be. In the meantime, pack your anti-ageing diet into no-cook snacks: peanut butter spread on multigrain toast; a bowl of walnuts and almonds; a wholemeal roll stuffed with tinned fresh salmon (drained, boned and mashed with a little vinegar) and a supermarket pack of watercress, or sticks of washed red pepper, courgettes and carrot to scoop up supermarket houmous.*

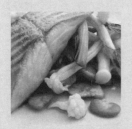
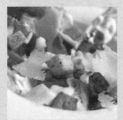
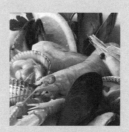

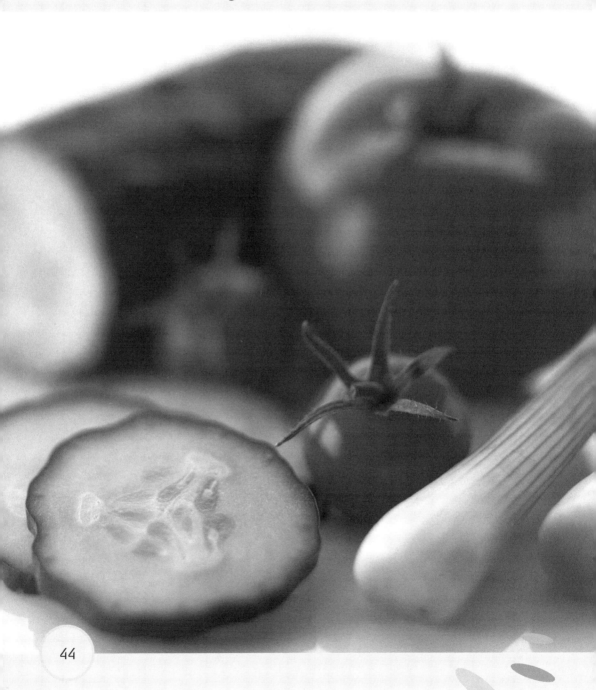

9

The veggie question

Studies show that vegetarians live longer and suffer less heart disease and cancer. Is it time to ditch the meat?

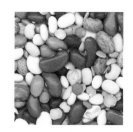

If you're a vegetarian, it's time to feel smug. You're already a winner when it comes to anti-ageing.

You can look forward to ten extra years of disease-free living than meat-eaters and you're 39% less likely to die from cancer. You're also 30% less likely to die of heart disease.

Anti-ageing scientists think meat doesn't do you many favours – and they point to the world's longest-lived communities to prove it. A famous study called the China Project highlighted the difference between mainly vegetarian Chinese from rural areas, who stay disease-free late into life, and their meat-eating urban counterparts who succumb to heart disease, stroke, osteoporosis, diabetes and cancer.

But hang on, you're thinking, if we're designed to munch plant food only, how come our cavemen ancestors ate meat? It's a good point. Trouble is, although the human race did evolve as omnivores, we now eat more meat in a week than our ancestors did in months. Obviously, this is partly because we no longer have to chase our meat with a spear before eating it. But it's also due to changes in farming

It's a myth that meat is the best source of protein – it's also found in some surprising foods, like brown rice for instance. Add a small tin of mixed beans (rinse them in a sieve under the tap first) to cooked, cooled brown rice and sprinkle with a few drops of sesame oil to taste. Garnish with fresh coriander and you've got a delicious, anti-ageing salad that contains all eight of the vital amino acids that protein supplies.

patterns that mean meat and dairy products are cheaper and more readily available than ever before.

If you're tucking into a burger right now, you may want to read the following paragraphs some other time. There's a theory that humans have a long colon, like a horse or cow, and a relatively slow food transit designed to break down grains and grasses. Too much meat introduced into the system literally rots before it reaches the end, releasing toxins into the bloodstream.

Dr Colin Campbell, chairman of the World Cancer Research Fund, believes 'animal protein is one of the most toxic nutrients there is' and that 'the vast majority, perhaps 80 to 90%, of all cancers, cardiovascular diseases and other forms of degenerative illness can be prevented, at least until very old age, simply by adopting a plant-based diet'. Still eating that burger? The theory is that animal fats are high in saturated fats which raise levels of bad (LDL) cholesterol, increasing the risk of heart disease. Vegetarians, by contrast, tend to eat a lot of plant-based foods which are high in disease-fighting antioxidants.

Most meat-eaters also eat too much protein (even those who aren't on the Atkins diet). According to the World Health Organization, we need around 35 g of protein a day, but the average meat-eating woman eats around 65 g and the average man, 90 g. We do need to eat some protein with every meal but you don't always have to add meat to ensure you get it. If your meal contains fish, lentils and beans, grains like rice, quinoa, and bulgar wheat, eggs, yogurt, cheese, nuts or seeds, you're probably already eating enough.

Pulses such as beans are not only a good source of protein – they're also high in disease-fighting antioxidants. Find out more on why they're vital to your diet at IDEA 6, *Upping the anti.*

Try another idea...

But what if you're a diehard meat fan who can't bear the thought of life without a Sunday roast? Don't despair – omnivores who eat above average amounts of fruit and vegetables can cut their risk of most cancers by 50–75%. And by increasing the amount of plant foods you eat, you'll probably find you naturally cut back on meat consumption.

'It always seems to me that man was not born to be a carnivore.'
Albert Einstein

Defining idea...

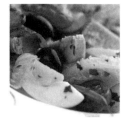
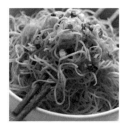
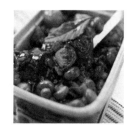

How did
it go?

Q   I'm a big bloke. Don't I need the protein from meat to keep me going?

A   *Are you heavier than the average male gorilla? They weigh in at nearly 400 kg (800 lb) which they happily sustain on a diet of vegetables, fruits and nuts. Many top sports nutritionists now recommend a vegetarian diet as the best way of building lean muscle tissue.*

Q   If I can't live without meat, which are the healthiest choices to opt for?

A   *Most nutritionists recommend switching from red meat to white meat, as that contains the less saturated fats. In Mediterranean countries red meat is seen as a treat for a couple of times a month. Skinless turkey breast is one of the leanest meats available, and it's also a good source of cancer-fighting selenium and zinc, which boosts the immune system. Chicken breast is also a good choice. If you can afford it, opt for organic meat which doesn't contain growth hormones and antibiotics. The very worst options are processed meats such as hot dogs, burgers and cured meats as they contain high amounts of nitrates which are thought to be carcinogenic. (In one study of 30,000 older women, those who ate a lot of hamburgers had twice the normal risk of certain kinds of cancer.) Char-grilled meat is also thought to be high in carcinogenic compounds known as HCAs – try stir-frying strips of meat instead.*

10

Time for an oil change?

Don't be afraid of fats – the right kind have a vital role to play in the anti-ageing process.

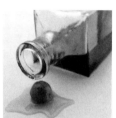

Confused about fat? Join the club. It's hardly surprising most of us don't quite know which way to turn, but it's not as complicated as you might think. It's all about getting the balance right.

In the last few years, we've cast off our fat phobia and joyfully indulged in an Atkins-fuelled fat frenzy, convinced we can feast on saturated fat with total impunity. But now the bubble has burst, rumours that diet guru Dr Atkins himself died obese are rife, and the company behind Atkins has been forced to temper its advice on fat, telling people to reign back on the amount of saturated fats and red meat they're consuming. So here's an easy four-step guide.

1. USE MORE OLIVE OIL

Olive oil lowers bad cholesterol and raises good, is essential for healthy cell formation and improves digestion. It's also packed with antioxidant vitamins A and E, as well as vitamins D and K, vital for strong bones. So it's no surprise that in

Here's an idea for you...

When shopping for olive oil, look for 'extra virgin'. It means the oil is pressed from olives that are not damaged, bruised or subjected to adverse temperatures or too much air, or that have had additional treatment such as heat or blending with other oils. What is simply termed olive oil is often a blend of lesser-quality refined oils with some virgin oil added to give the right balance of flavour. Extra virgin olive oil, however, has the highest concentration of cancer-fighting antioxidants.

those Mediterranean communities where people live the longest, where rates of heart disease are astonishingly low, olive oil is used with abandon – it's poured over salads, used instead of butter on bread and drizzled over cooked vegetables. Some anti-ageing experts say olive oil is the only oil they have in the house – they use it for all cooking and dressings.

2. CUT BACK ON SOLID FATS

A diet high in saturates can raise levels of LDL ('bad') blood cholesterol and increase the risk of heart disease. Saturated fats tend to be solid at room temperature (think butter, margarine, lard, suet and dripping) or come from animal sources (meat, eggs, milk, cheese, yogurt), although two vegetable oils, coconut and palm oil, are also high in saturates. Limit this to small amounts such as a knob of butter on vegetables or some cheese crumbled on a salad. But don't try to cut it out altogether – it's the best source of fat-soluble vitamins A and D, vital for healthy skin, teeth, hair, bones and vision.

3. KEEP POLYUNSATURATED OILS TO A MINIMUM

Polyunsaturated vegetable oils have been sold as a healthy choice but anti-ageing experts keep them at arm's length. While polyunsaturates from natural sources such as nuts and fish are essential for a healthy heart and brain, once they are processed to become oils, their natural antioxidants are removed. The end result can be toxic – they form lipid oxidation products (LOPs) in the body which can attack the arteries. Keep soy, peanut and corn oils to a minimum (often these are just labelled 'vegetable oils'). Sunflower oil is a better choice as it contains higher levels of the antioxidant vitamin E, but the best choice of all, for cooking and dressings, is olive oil.

The oil in many fish is vital to any anti-ageing diet. Find out why at IDEA 11, *Get hooked on fish*.

Try another idea...

4. AVOID TRANS FATS

Trans fats are a form of polyunsaturates that are made when oils are processed by hydrogenation. This is used by the food industry to provide moistness in foods such as cakes, biscuits, pastries, pies and sausages. It's also used to stop margarines melting at room temperature and is found in many polyunsaturated margarines marketed as 'healthy'. But studies have shown that trans fats raise levels of LDL cholesterol in the body to a greater extent than saturated fats, while simultaneously reducing levels of 'good' HDL cholesterol. Around 30,000 heart-attack deaths a year in the US can be attributed to high levels of trans fats in the diet. Trans fats have also been linked with free radical damage to body cells that can lead to cancer and heart disease. Play safe by avoiding all products that contain trans fats – look for hydrogenated vegetable oil in the ingredients list. (It's also sometimes labelled as 'partially hydrogenated' or 'shortening'.)

'Spaghetti, a love of life and the odd bath in virgin olive oil.'
Sophia Loren's explanation for her youthful good looks at 70

Defining idea...

51

How did
it go?

Q   **So how do I know if I'm eating too much fat – good or bad?**

A   *For optimal anti-ageing, if you consume 2000 calories a day, you should eat no more than 70 g of fat, including no more than 20 g of saturates or trans fats. You'd get 70 g of fat in a day if you included a tablespoon peanut butter plus one large egg, plus a small chunk of brie, plus a blueberry muffin, plus a handful of sunflower seeds, plus a small mackerel fillet and a low-fat yogurt. But don't get hung up on trying to work out exactly how much you're eating – base the bulk of your diet on natural foods like fruit and vegetables, nuts and seeds, fish and meat, and you'll naturally eat the right amount of fat.*

Q   **But all fat makes you fat, right?**

A   *Not so – some might actually help you slim because they help you feel full for longer. In one study, two groups ate 1200 calories a day, but one group ate 35% of these calories from foods containing monounsaturated fats. Both groups lost about 5 kg (over 11 lb) in the first six weeks. But eighteen months later twice as many in the higher fat group had maintained their weight loss. In another study, people who added a snack of 500 calories in peanuts every day for eight weeks on top of their existing calorie intake didn't gain any weight. The researchers believe that the fats in peanuts may raise the metabolism, and also help reduce food consumption throughout the day. Walnuts, pecans and almonds may have the same effect.*

11

Get hooked on fish

Simply opening a tin of sardines can stave off wrinkles (if you eat the sardines)...

Your grandmother was talking sense after all – fish really is good for your brain and a daily dose of cod liver oil will keep you strong and healthy.

But what she may not have realised is that fish can also fend off ageing and help you look and feel younger. It all comes down to some special fatty acids found in fish called omega-3s. These oils are vital for the functioning of every cell in our bodies, and yet our bodies cannot make them – we have to get them from food. Ready for some long words? Two particularly valuable omega-3s are docosahexaenoic acid (DHA) and eicosapentaenoic acid (EPA) and you'll find high levels in salmon, herrings, sardines, pilchards, mackerel, tuna and trout.

A recent best-selling book recommended eating salmon three times a day instead of having a facelift. Converts swore that it reduced wrinkles. Omega-3 fatty acids do contain a chemical that stimulates nerve function and encourages the muscles under the skin to contract and tighten. But you don't have to eat fish as often as that to help you *feel* younger for longer.

Here's an idea for you...

Stuck for easy fish ideas? What about fresh salmon, grilled or poached in a little milk and garnished with fresh dill or parsley? Whole mackerel is a great fish to cook on a barbecue or try them stuffed with lemon chunks and herbs and baked in foil for a stylish dinner. Or try adding ready-to-eat smoked trout fillets to a salad, giving a lunch that's high in cancer-fighting selenium as well as omega-3s. Tins are also good – add a tin of anchovies to tomato-based pasta sauces or use as a pizza topping. Or mash a tin of sardines, herring or pilchards onto multigrain toast for a speedy snack or simple supper.

Take the Inuit. Did you know they don't have a word in their language for heart attack because it's so rare among them? This is thought to be thanks to their diet – and some doctors are now recommending that we copy it. But if you don't fancy whale or seal blubber all winter, don't worry – you get the same benefits from eating the fish that whales and seals eat: salmon, herring, anchovies, mackerel and tuna. The omega-3 fatty acids 'calm down' the artery walls, as well as reducing production of bad LDL cholesterol, raising levels of good HDL cholesterol, lowering blood pressure and reducing irregular heart beats.

Thanks to reams of other studies, we now know that these valuable oils play a role in staving off stroke and breast cancer, fighting asthma and protecting joints. There's scientific research to back up what our ancestors knew by instinct – that fish is good for the brain. One study found that older people who eat fish or seafood once a week have a significantly lower risk of developing dementia.

Defining idea...

'Fish, to taste good, must swim three times: in water, in butter and in wine.'
Polish proverb

Omega-3s work best as part of a double act with another group of essential oils called omega-6s, found in vegetable oils such as sunflower, soy, hemp and linseed, which are important for lowering blood cholesterol and supporting the skin. Thanks to the widespread use of sunflower oil in food processing, few of us are deficient in omega-6s, but at the same time, intake of omega-3s has dropped by more than half (we don't eat so much fish and tend to go for low fat varieties such as cod and haddock rather than herring and mackerel). Scientists now believe that too many omega-6s in the diet can undo the good work of omega-3s. To redress the balance, try to cut down on fried and processed foods and margarines and eat more oily fish – aim for a minimum of twice a week.

Omega-3s aren't the only fats that are good for you. Monounsaturates are also effective in staving off ageing. See IDEA 10, *Time for an oil change?*

Try another idea...

Q   What about the recent news stories about pollutants in fish?

How did it go?

A   *You're right to be concerned. News reports have described high levels of mercury, a naturally occurring mineral, which is poisonous in large amounts, in some fish. Pregnant women have been advised to avoid large fish such as marlin, swordfish, tuna and shark (the bigger the fish, the more pollutants is the theory). However, high levels of mercury have not been found in fish such as mackerel, herring, pilchard, sardine, trout or salmon, so it's safe to eat these two or three times a week. More recently, we've read reports of high levels of cancer-causing pollutants such as dioxins and PCBs (polychlorinated biphenyls) in farmed salmon, but it's still uncertain whether*

55

these contaminants are at high enough levels to affect human health. Most nutritionists say that the benefits of eating oily fish two or three times a week far outweigh the risks. And it's not all bad news – a recent study found that the level of dioxins in oily fish has declined by 50% over the past three years, the result of environmental clean-ups stretching back to the 1970s which are only now showing their effects.

Q **I'm sorry – I just can't stomach fish. What else contains omega-3s?**

A *Although the evidence we have to date about the benefits of essential fatty acids in cutting down heart disease and stroke and improving brain function has centred on two fatty acids – EPA and DHA – found only in oily fish, studies in the future may show a similar benefit from vegetarian sources. Good vegetarian sources of omega-3s are linseeds (flaxseeds) in oil, seed or supplement form, walnuts and pumpkin seeds (try adding a handful of flaxseeds to soups, stews or salads every day). Plus, the food industry has now added omega-3s to some eggs and orange juices. You can also opt for a fish oil supplement – studies suggest that supplements high in omega-3s (look for DHA and EPA on the ingredients label) can provide the bulk of the benefits associated with eating oily fish. One note of caution – fish oil is rich in vitamin E which may affect warfarin treatment so always check with your doctor before taking the supplement if you're on warfarin.*

12

Have a cuppa

Now here's something we can all do to improve our chances of living a longer, healthier life – drink a cup of tea. Put the kettle on!

It's almost too good to be true. Just by curling up in a chair with a cup of tea, you're lowering your blood pressure, fighting cancer, osteoporosis, heart disease and wrinkles.

Tea is one of our most ancient drinks but only recently has research revealed its remarkable anti-ageing powers. It's packed with flavonoids, disease-fighting compounds that reduce the damaging effects of free radicals on your body's cells. Tea contains a particularly potent variety called catechins which have been shown to be more powerful antioxidants than vitamins C and E in laboratory tests. But they're just one of tea's nearly 4000 phytochemicals which are thought to work synergistically to fight disease.

It seems there's no end to the ways that tea can help you live longer. It can lower your risk of having a heart attack and stave off cancer. In one extraordinary study, green and black tea rubbed onto precancerous lesions reduced the growth of the

Here's how to get the most from your cuppa. Tea should be made with freshly boiled, but not boiling water, which can reduce its antioxidant capacity. So let the water sit in the kettle for a minute before pouring it on the tea. Allow the tea bag to steep for three to five minutes to bring out its catechins. Then give it a good squeeze – this can double the amount of flavonoids released. Green and white teas taste best drunk without milk. If you prefer to add milk to black tea, go ahead – a recent review of tea studies suggests it doesn't affect the health benefits.

cells. In mice, tea has also been shown to slow the development of lung tumours and colon cancer. It also keeps your prostate healthy. Men in East Asia who drink lots of green tea have much lower rates of prostate cancer than men in the rest of the world, thought to be due to green tea's antioxidants.

Tea also protects your joints. Researchers have found that two compounds in green tea block the enzyme that destroys cartilage. Other studies have shown that tea can even play a role in strengthening your bones and reducing the risk of hip fractures. And it's good for your teeth – it fights the bacteria that cause gum disease and contains fluoride which helps fend off decay.

It also reduces skin damage. The compounds in green tea fight DNA damage induced by ultraviolet light – the source of skin ageing (and skin cancer). It's why green tea extract is a favourite ingredient in anti-ageing cosmetics.

And just in case you're still not sold on the idea, if not already in the process of making a cup – tea may even help you lose weight! A preliminary study has found that an extract from green tea may help with weight loss by speeding up fat metabolism.

But what's the best type of tea to opt for? It all comes from a single plant (*Camellia sinensis*), but differences in processing after harvesting produce different 'colours' of tea. And it seems

For more ways to boost your antioxidant levels, see IDEA 6, *Upping the anti.*

Try another idea...

that while all true teas (herbal or fruit teas aren't true teas) have health benefits, some have more than others. The classic cup of black tea, usually drunk with milk, is made up of leaves that have been left to ferment after harvesting, which darkens them and allows them to develop a stronger flavour. Green tea is much more lightly processed than black and contains slightly more flavonoids than black (316 mg per cup compared with 268 mg). It also contains a higher percentage of catechins. Recently, there's been big excitement over white tea – it's been hailed as the most antioxidant-rich tea of all. It's made from very small buds picked in the early spring, before they have opened. It's the rarest tea in the world, produced on a very limited scale in China and Sri Lanka – which is reflected in the price.

But green, black or white will all give you a powerful antioxidant boost if you drink around four cups a day. Which colour you opt for is a matter of taste, although many people prefer the 'kick' of black tea at breakfast and the lighter, more refreshing taste of green or white throughout the day. Adding four or more cups a day is probably one of the cheapest, easiest and most enjoyable ways to fight ageing.

'If you are cold, tea will warm you. If you are heated, it will cool you. If you are depressed, it will cheer you. If you are excited, it will calm you.'
William Gladstone, nineteenth-century British Prime Minister

Defining idea...

How did it go?

Q **If tea contains so many flavonoids, does it count as one of my 'five-a-day' fruit and vegetable portions?**

A *In theory, yes – a couple of cups of tea have as many flavonoids as twenty glasses of apple juice. But fruit and vegetables also contain essential vitamins and fibre that you won't get in a cuppa. So add your four or more cups a day to a diet based on lots of vegetables and fruit for maximum effect. And while research is showing us that tea does have incredible protective powers, it's not a magic bullet – it can't undo the damage caused by a poor diet, smoking or too much alcohol.*

Q **My coffee shop sells 'tea latte' – does this count as real tea?**

A *Tea latte is basically chai (rhymes with 'pie'), black tea made with warm, sweetened milk and lots of spices such as cardamom, cinnamon, ginger, cloves and pepper. Sold for next to nothing by street traders in India, it's been hijacked by trendy coffee bars in the West, given a new name and a huge price hike. You will get some antioxidant benefits from this drink as it's made from real tea, but if you're watching your weight, stick to regular tea – it has far fewer calories.*

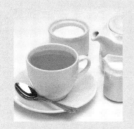
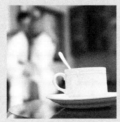

13

The good news about booze

Here's some news to drink to – people who have two to three small glasses of red wine a day live longer than people who don't.

Scientists are finally coming up with an explanation for what people in France, Spain, Italy and Greece have known for centuries — that a couple of small glasses of wine a day keep you young and healthy.

While it's well-established that moderate drinking can fend off heart disease, an exciting new study suggests it may actually fight the ageing process itself. This was carried out by scientists at Harvard Medical School, who found that the potent antioxidant called resveratrol found in red wine could extend the life of yeast in a laboratory experiment by 60–80%. Although we've known for some time that resveratrol is a great ally in the battle against damaging free radicals, what got the scientists so excited was that this study showed it might have another, quite different effect. They think that it stimulates special enzymes in the body called sirtuins that prevent cell death.

Here's an idea for you...

A simple way to cut down on your wine consumption without feeling deprived is to buy some traditionally sized, 125 ml wine glasses to use at home. They may not be as trendy as the bucket-sized glasses now in vogue, but they'll help you keep track of your units. One of these glasses is around one unit and most people say they sip their wine more slowly if it's in a smaller glass. Always ask for a 125 ml glass in bars or restaurants too.

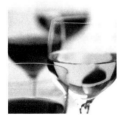

The only other way this has been made to happen has been in studies of very restricted calorie diets. And, given the choice, most people would rather drink more red wine than starve themselves!

Although more research is needed to find out if red wine has the same effect on human cells, it fits in with other studies that give moderate wine drinking the thumbs up. According to a recent report the more wine you drink, the lower your risk of death – not just from coronary heart disease but from all causes of death, including cancer.

The French habit of drinking a glass of wine with meals is thought to explain the so-called French paradox: their high intake of saturated fat but low rate of heart disease. In fact, regular wine drinking is credited by cardiologists for the low rate of heart disease generally in Mediterranean countries. It's thought that red wine interferes with the production of a body chemical which clogs up arteries and increases the risk of a heart attack. And when given to cancer-prone mice in another study, red wine increased lifespan by 50%, thought to be due to the anti-cancer properties of two powerful flavonoids.

But it goes without saying that moderation is the key. The proof that too much booze speeds up the ageing process can usually be found propping up a bar! Too much alcohol *increases* your risk of heart disease and cancer (not to mention liver disease). Plus, as anyone who's ever had a hangover can testify by simply looking in the mirror, too much alcohol has a severely dehydrating – and ageing – effect on the skin. It's essential to stick to two or three small drinks a night, stay within the recommended weekly limits (21 units for men and 14 for women) and have at least two alcohol-free days a week. Try to drink while you're eating food and sip water as well. Opt for the deepest red wines made from these grapes to get maximum flavonoids in every glass: Merlot, Cabernet Sauvignon, or Pinot Noir. Stick to these simple rules and drinking can be one of the most enjoyable ways to stave off ageing. Cheers!

Teetotal? Don't worry – olive oil has similar anti-ageing effects to red wine. For more reasons why an oil change might stave off ageing, see IDEA 10, *Time for an oil change?*

Try another idea...

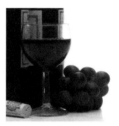

'Wine is constant proof that God loves us and loves to see us happy.'
Benjamin Franklin

Defining idea...

How did it go?

Q **Great! I got so carried away I finished the whole bottle. But I'll still be under 21 units if I don't drink again all week, so that's OK, isn't it?**

A *Only if you want to speed up ageing. Depending on how strong it is, the average bottle of wine contains between 7 and 10 units. Downing that much at once is classed as binge drinking, which has been linked with an increased risk of stroke, hypertension, some cancers and heart disease. In fact, a new report points out that up to 40% of men's drinking sessions now technically qualify as binge drinking and that accounts for up to 22,000 premature deaths each year. So next time aim for just a couple of glasses and save the rest for another night.*

Q **Red wine's not my favourite tipple. Can I get the same effect from white wine, beer or a gin and tonic?**

A *Good news – studies have linked all moderate alcohol intake drinking (around two small drinks a day) with a lower risk of heart attacks, stroke, hypertension, diabetes and dementia – one theory is that social drinkers tend to have lower stress levels and a better support network than non-drinkers, which helps them recover quickly from physical and mental setbacks. And a new study from the Netherlands has found that people who drink beer with dinner for several weeks have lower levels of homocysteine – which can age the arteries and increase the risk of heart disease in high levels – than people who drink wine or gin. But you'll only find large amounts of resveratrol, the powerful antioxidant that's been shown to lower the risk of cancer in laboratory tests, in red wine. You'd be wise to make this your main tipple.*

14

The joy of soy

Soy beans are mini powerhouses, full of disease-fighting nutrients.

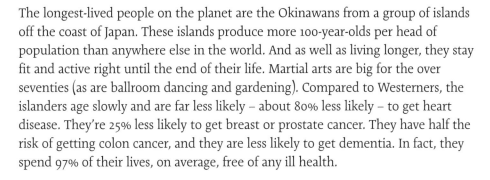

They contain anti-cancer compounds, are good for your heart and can help with the menopause. They can even taste nice, too!

The longest-lived people on the planet are the Okinawans from a group of islands off the coast of Japan. These islands produce more 100-year-olds per head of population than anywhere else in the world. And as well as living longer, they stay fit and active right until the end of their life. Martial arts are big for the over seventies (as are ballroom dancing and gardening). Compared to Westerners, the islanders age slowly and are far less likely – about 80% less likely – to get heart disease. They're 25% less likely to get breast or prostate cancer. They have half the risk of getting colon cancer, and they are less likely to get dementia. In fact, they spend 97% of their lives, on average, free of any ill health.

According to a 25-year study of the islanders, it's largely down to one thing – their love of soy. Okinawans eat about three ounces a day, in miso, tofu, soy sauce and soy milk.

Here's an idea for you...

It's time to face your fear of tofu. OK, it's white, flabby and flavourless – but cooked correctly it can be delicious. The key is marinating it before cooking. First, pour off the water it's stored in and press with a clean tea towel until dry. Cut into cubes or strips, then marinate in 4 tablespoons of soy or sunflower oil, 4 tablespoons of lemon juice, 3 tablespoons of soy sauce, 2 teaspoons of honey and a tablespoon of grated ginger for an hour. Remove from the marinade and stir-fry in a wok for 2–3 minutes until brown. Add finely chopped vegetables such as carrots, spring onions, red pepper, mushrooms and Chinese leaves, and the rest of the marinade. Stir-fry for 4–5 minutes, then serve.

But the soy story doesn't end there. In mainland Japan, where the diet is also high in soy products, the breast cancer rate is the lowest in the world. And in soy-eating countries like Korea, the rate of breast cancer is between a sixth and a tenth of the rate in the West. It seems that women with a soy-rich diet have breast tissue which is less dense than women with low soy diets – and a higher density of breast tissue has been linked to a higher risk of breast cancer.

Soy beans are thought to contain around six different anti-cancer compounds, the most powerful of all being isoflavones. Isoflavones block oestrogen, a hormone linked with increased risk of breast cancer, and testosterone, which is linked with prostate cancer. One isoflavone, known as genistein, has been shown to actually turn cancer cells back into normal ones. It may also cut off blood vessels from existing tumours, stopping their growth. A sudden reduction in the amount of soy in the diet is thought to be the reason why Japanese men who emigrate to work in America have high rates of prostate cancer. One theory is that the cancers were present before they left for America, but they were held in check by soy in the diet. Once soy consumption goes down, the cancers spring into life.

Soy is also good for your heart. It lowers levels of bad (LDL) cholesterol and raises levels of good (HDL) cholesterol, helping to keep the arteries clear. One study found that adding soy to the diet dropped the cholesterol levels of people at risk from heart disease by 26%. Other studies have shown it can help relieve menopausal symptoms.

Isoflavone-rich foods such as soy are great for strengthening bones. For more ways, see IDEA 44, Bone up.

Try another idea...

Soy's got a bit of a hippie-dippie reputation and if you're allergic to health-food stores it can be a bit off-putting. But it's come a long way recently – and so have health-food stores – and you can now buy soy products in most supermarkets. Look out for tofu (made from soy bean curd), soy milk, soy sauce, miso soup, and whole soy beans. Here are some easy ways to eat more.

1. Use soy milk on your breakfast cereal in the morning.
2. Look out for edamame in Asian grocers' – fresh soy beans in their pods. Simply lightly steam then pop the beans from their pods and eat.
3. Ask for your coffee-shop cappuccino to be made with soy milk.
4. Add tinned soy beans (from health-food stores) when making soups.
5. Look for soy yogurt and ice cream in supermarkets for dessert.
6. Whizz up soy milk, a couple of ounces of silken tofu and a banana or handful of berries to make a fruit smoothie for breakfast.
7. Use soy mince instead of regular mince in dishes such as spaghetti bolognese.

'Did you ever see the customers in health-food stores? They are pale, skinny people. In a steak house, you see robust, ruddy people. They're dying, of course, but they look terrific.'
Bill Cosby

Defining idea...

8. Opt for breads that contain soy, such as Burgen soya and linseed loaf.
9. Use miso paste (a fermented mash of crushed soy beans) instead of stock cubes.
10. Add a dash of soy sauce instead of salt when you're cooking.

How did it go?

Q   I recently read that soy can be bad for you. Is this true?

A   *There has been negative publicity recently about the amount of soy used to bulk out foods such as sausages and pies by the food processing industry. It's been suggested that men eating a lot of processed food could be getting enough phyto-oestrogens to have a negative effect on their fertility. Plus, when soy oil is heated at high temperatures during food processing, it becomes a dangerous trans fat. But if the bulk of your diet comes from fresh foods, eating too much soy is not something to lose any sleep over.*

Q   So how much soy do I have to eat exactly?

A   *The long-lived Okinawans eat it twice a day. But you don't have to have it with every meal to get the desired effect. Just 50 g (2 oz) a day – one soy yogurt or some soy milk on your cereal at breakfast – should have an effect, or 100 g (4 oz) every two days.*

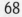

15

Porridge power

Starting the day with a humble bowl of porridge can add years to your life.

Porridge is on the verge of megastardom. It's about to become the trendiest consumable since coffee shops reinvented coffee. Anyone who wants to live longer should make it a part of their diet.

It's shaking off its image as a dull but worthy way of filling yourself up for little money. In the States customers are already queuing up at a chain of cafés called Cereality to buy takeaway cartons of the stuff. Whether we'll all be nipping out for a quick porridge soon instead of a burger remains to be seen, but we should definitely eat more.

A daily bowl of porridge sustained the ancient Scots through hours of marauding. They knew that if you started the day with porridge, you didn't feel hungry for hours. Now we know that porridge does a lot more than just give you energy.

Here's an idea for you... **There is a lot of mystique about making porridge but it actually couldn't be easier. There's really one thing to remember – stir! Start with good quality medium-ground porridge oats (rather than rolled oats). For two people, you'll need one pint of water (or half water and half milk for a creamier taste) and two and a half rounded tablespoons of oats. Bring the water (or water and milk) to the boil in a non-stick pan. Slowly pour the oatmeal into the boiling liquid, stirring vigorously with a wooden spoon all the time. Keep stirring until it has returned to the boil again, reduce the heat, cover the pan and simmer very gently for fifteen minutes, stirring frequently. Add a pinch of salt and simmer, stirring until it's thickened up.**

Porridge oats are packed with a rich source of cancer-fighting phyto-oestrogens, and the antioxidant polyphenols. They contain a particularly powerful antioxidant called ferulic acid which seems to actually stop certain cancer-promoting compounds in their tracks.

Start the day with porridge, and you're also doing your heart a big favour. Scientists have found that porridge contains avenanthramides – chemicals that stop blood cells sticking to artery walls, preventing the fatty deposits that cause heart disease. And a daily serving of oats can improve blood pressure control and stop or reduce the need for blood pressure medication by half. Eating oats also reduces cholesterol levels.

If you're not worried about your heart, then what about your waistline? Porridge only masquerades as stodgy comfort food – in truth, it's the nearest thing we've got to a magic diet pill. People who eat wholegrain-based breakfasts such as porridge every day are a third less likely to be obese compared to those who skip the meal. The researchers believe that eating porridge first thing in the morning may help to stabilise blood sugar levels, which regulate appetite and energy. They also suggest that people who eat oats for breakfast are less likely to be hungry during the rest of the day

Not having enough fibre in your diet can take years off your life. Find out what to do about this at IDEA 16, *Foods to lose.*

Try another idea...

and are, therefore, less likely to overeat. It's thought that slowly digested foods such as porridge might cut the risk of developing diabetes, by absorbing sugar from the gut and cutting the need for large quantities of insulin to be released.

Finally, eat a bowl of porridge and you'll be boosting your gut flora (you know, the bugs in your digestive tract that keep food moving through the system). We've always known oats were good for keeping you regular, but now scientists have discovered they're a good source of probiotics, food for your body's good bacteria. The more food these bacteria have, the more they multiply – and the better they are at fending off disease-causing toxic bacteria. The end result? A strengthened immune system – all from a humble bowl of oats.

'The healsome porritch, chief of Scotia's food.'
Robert Burns

Defining idea...

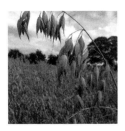 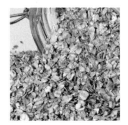

How did
it go?

Q I really hate porridge. Can I eat something else?

A *Yes – you can experience the benefits of porridge by boosting the fibre in the diet generally. You could start with a wholegrain breakfast cereal or wholegrain toast. Look for the word 'whole' in the ingredients list and a fibre content of at least 3 g per serving in the panel on nutritional information. Then throughout the day, opt for wholegrain rice and pasta instead of white varieties, and eat at least two servings of fresh fruit and five of vegetables. Try snacking on oatcakes – delicious with low-fat cream cheese. How about adding handfuls of oatmeal to other dishes such as soup, or to homemade fish cakes? And one cheap and easy way to boost the fibre in your diet is to buy a bag of wheatgerm from a health-food store and add it to soups and casseroles. It's a great source of omega-3 fatty acids as well as fibre.*

Q I made some porridge and it was like wallpaper paste. Does it always taste like that?

A *The secret's in the added extras. Traditionally, it was served with a good dollop of double cream or sprinkling of brown sugar. But if you're not going to burn off those extra calories with hours of marauding, then opt for a couple of tablespoons of natural bio-yogurt and a pinch of cinnamon or grated nutmeg, or a drizzle of honey. Or try throwing in a handful of frozen mixed berries or some sultanas halfway through cooking, or serving it topped with dried fruit – the long-lived Hunza people of the Himalayas swear by hot porridge with dried apricots and almonds.*

16
Foods to lose

Meet the four nutritional no-nos that speed up the ageing process.

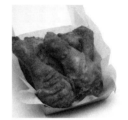

Here's a simple equation for you — to live longer, eat less food but take in more nutrients.

Your body needs a wide range of micronutrients to fight the ageing process, but it doesn't need excess calories so the key is to make every meal count. You can't go wrong if you base your diet on fruits, vegetables, wholegrains, nuts, olive oil and fish. But there are also foods to avoid. Here are your main anti-ageing enemies.

REFINED SUGAR

Eat too much sugar and you'll get more wrinkles. Sugar can react with proteins in the body, a chemical reaction known as glycosylation. As blood sugar levels increase, so does the rate of glycosylation. In the blood vessels, glycosylation can cause hardening of the arteries and kidney damage. But glycosylation in the skin disrupts the connective tissue in a process known as cross-linking. The effect is skin that's less elastic, more prone to wrinkles. The key to limiting glycosylation is to avoid blood sugar peaks, usually caused by foods that contain added sugars (look for

Here's an idea for you...

Can't get through the day without a sweet treat? Then have some chocolate. Yes, that's right, chocolate is an anti-ageing food. Chocolate eaters live longer than non-chocolate eaters, if they eat the right kind. Dark chocolate with a high (70%) cocoa content is an excellent source of flavonoids and actually provides more antioxidants than many fruits and vegetables. It also provides more calories, so eaten in excess you'll pile on the pounds. But a few squares two or three times a week will give you an antioxidant boost that will also satisfy a sweet tooth.

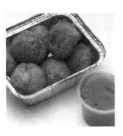

glucose, sucrose, fructose and corn syrup on labels). Peaks in blood sugar levels also trigger the 'fight or flight' hormones – adrenaline and cortisone – which suppress the body's immune system. Too much sugar in the bloodstream on a regular basis can also damage the kidneys, nerves, eyesight, immune system and arteries. So have sweet things as occasional treats and opt for fruit and desserts based on natural yogurt instead.

REFINED CARBOHYDRATES

Low-carb dieters who believe carbohydrates are the work of the devil have got it half right. Wholegrain carbohydrates are made from every part of the grain and have been shown to lower the risk of heart disease, stroke, diabetes, obesity and certain cancers. But once these grains are refined, it's a very different story. Refined carbs have had all their powerful nutrients – antioxidants and phytonutrients – stripped away, leaving foodstuffs that provide energy in the form of calories but very little else. Refined carbohydrates are converted easily into glucose by the body and can cause peaks in blood sugar and the release of large amounts of insulin. Excesses of this hormone have been linked with major age-related conditions including Type 2 diabetes, heart disease and some forms of cancer. Use wholegrain bread, flour, pasta, rice and sweet potatoes instead.

The wrong kinds of fat can also speed up the ageing process. Find out how at IDEA 10, *Time for an oil change?*

Try another idea...

FAST FOOD

Fast food chains are spending a lot of money to convince us that our health won't be affected by eating junk. Remember what happened to film director Morgan Spurlock who ate nothing but McDonald's for one month for his movie *Supersize Me*. The first week he put on nearly 5 kg (10 lb). After a month, he'd added a total of just over 11 kg (25 lb). His cholesterol level rose by 65 points (a third higher than when he started). Most shocking of all, his doctor – who begged the film-maker to abandon the experiment after three weeks – concluded that his fast food intake was causing serious liver damage. In the film's postscript, Spurlock noted that it took him fourteen months to return to his former physical condition. So avoid burgers, kebabs and chips if you want to live longer.

PROCESSED FOODS

Packaged meals seem like the perfect solution to busy lifestyles. Base your diet on them and you'll almost certainly speed up the ageing process, simply because you'll be consuming far

'Why pay for food that's going to age you and make you fat?'
Dr Michael Roizen, US anti-ageing guru

Defining idea...

too much salt. We need some salt to regulate fluid balance, but too much causes high blood pressure, a risk factor for strokes and heart attacks. Adults need around a gram a day (about half a teaspoon) and the healthy maximum is 6 g. We're currently getting almost double this a day, on average. Cutting back to the healthy max has been estimated to prevent 22% of strokes and 16% of heart attacks. Only 20% of the salt we consume is added during cooking or at the table; the rest – 80% – is added during food processing. When reading labels on foods, remember that a single gram of sodium is equivalent to 2.55 g of salt. Try to eat as many unprocessed foods as possible and look out for 'hidden salt' in bread, cereals and stock cubes.

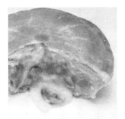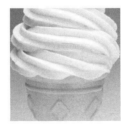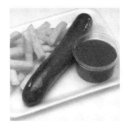

Q **I've done a week without fast food and I've never felt worse. Is this normal?**

How did it go?

A *Fast food is as addictive as heroin, according to one researcher who found that high-fat foods stimulated opioids or pleasure chemicals in the brains of rats. So you may be suffering withdrawal symptoms, especially if you're used to eating fast food for comfort. Stick with a wholegrain diet high in fresh produce and you'll soon notice a different kind of high – a natural one that comes from health and vitality.*

Q **I have to eat out a lot so what are the most anti-ageing foods I can choose?**

A *Simple – think of what you'd eat at home and try to order it in a restaurant or takeaway. In a sandwich bar, ask for wholegrain bread and boost your omega-3s by opting for poached salmon (with no mayo) and salad leaves. Italian restaurants are easy – just opt for lycopene-boosting, tomato-based sauce, but don't eat all the pasta; a healthy serving is around the size of a fist. Chinese takeaways are a great opportunity to eat soy by choosing tofu with stir-fried vegetables. And believe it or not, the healthiest option of all is the kebab house. You can fill up on a salad pitta, stuffed with antioxidant-packed raw veg like grated onion, carrots and cabbage, dressed with chilli sauce, yogurt or houmous.*

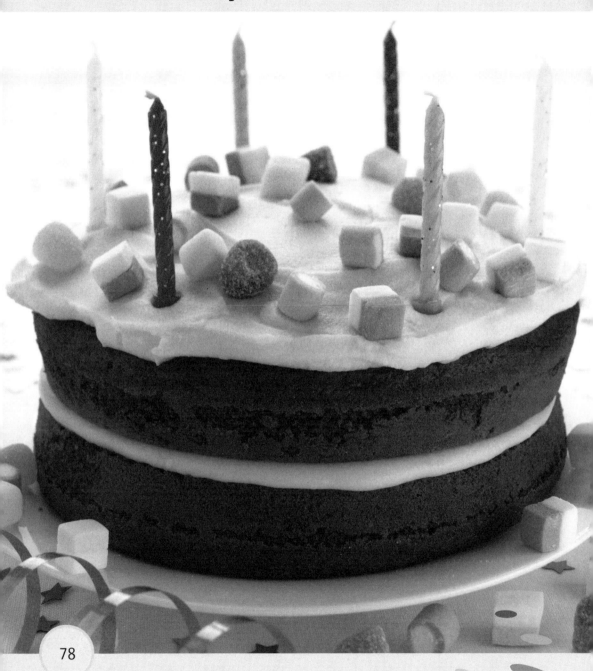

17

Less cake, more birthdays?

Reducing your calorie intake can stave off ageing and reduce your chances of getting serious diseases. But how can you do it without feeling deprived?

If you want to live longer, practise hara hachi. It means stopping eating when you're 80% full. By doing so, you naturally cut 10–40% of calories from your diet.

It's a tip from the longest-living people on earth, the inhabitants of the island of Okinawa in Japan. Starving has never been good for longevity. But eating just enough, rather than too many, calories can help you live younger for longer. In fact, reducing calorie intake is the one thing that anti-ageing scientists can definitely say has an impact on lifespan at present. In lab experiments, mice live twice as long as normal if their daily calorie intake is halved. They also stay younger for longer (apparently it's perfectly possible to tell if a mouse is young for its age).

Here's an idea for you...

No good at mental arithmetic? Then ditch calorie counting and use this 'handy' guide to portion control instead.
- **a portion of meat or fish: the size and thickness of your palm.**
- **a portion of hard cheese: the length and width of your thumb.**
- **a portion of cereal: the size of your fist.**
- **a portion of vegetables: two cupped handfuls.**
- **a portion of cooked rice, pasta or potatoes: one cupped handful.**
- **a portion of jacket potato: the size of your fist.**
- **a portion of butter or margarine: the tip of your thumb (from the knuckle).**

The theory is that calorie restriction inhibits the creation of free radicals, those destructive particles that harm genes and proteins. Others speculate that a reduced calorie diet catapults the body into a survival mode that retards the ageing process.

In the States converts to calorie restriction for longer life call themselves 'cronies', and they say the benefits are low blood pressure and cholesterol levels, abundant energy and an imperviousness to colds and flu. Cronies eat around 1400 calories a day if they're female and 1800 if they're male (compare this to what the average woman eats – around 2000 calories a day – and the average man, around 2600). The Okinawans eat around 1500 calories a day.

Reducing your calorie intake by a third is probably worth considering if you're overweight. But do get advice from a qualified dietician if you're restricting calories and you have any health problems, to make sure you don't miss out on any vital nutrients. The key to success is making sure every single one of those calories delivers a maximum nutrient punch. That means saying goodbye to nutritionally empty fast food, processed food, alcohol, sweets and cakes and basing the bulk of your diet on wholegrains, pulses, fruit and vegetables. A high-nutrient, low-calorie diet both limits the amounts of free radicals generated *and* provides large amounts of antioxidants that neutralise the effects of free radicals on the body.

Not sure what foods you should be concentrating on? Find out what to cut out at IDEA 16, *Foods to lose.*

Try another idea...

The latest research has found that you can also fend off ageing with intermittent fasts. It's thought that fasting produces mild stress which triggers the production of substances known as stress-resistance proteins, which are resistant to disease. In addition, it increases the production of a brain chemical which promotes learning, memory, and the growth and survival of nerve cells.

You can get these effects by cutting back to 500–600 calories one day a week or fortnight – by just having one meal on that day. But it doesn't mean the rest of the week can be a junk food binge; that would undermine all your efforts. Try to base the bulk of your diet on fruit, vegetables, wholegrains, nuts, soy, olive oil, lean meats, fish and low-fat dairy products.

'Hara hachi bu.'
Okinawan saying meaning 'eat until you're only eight parts full.'

Defining idea...

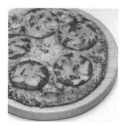 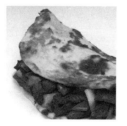

Q   Do I really have to feel hungry for the rest of my life?

A   *Definitely not – it's hard to function if you're constantly thinking of food. Reduce your intake by no more than 200–300 calories a day. You could start by eating normal food but simply leaving a small portion of it on the plate (and if you switch to eating more wholegrains you'll feel fuller anyway). As you get used to eating smaller portions and your stomach shrinks, you shouldn't feel hungry. But if you also feel light-headed, weak and lethargic, you've overdone it – eat more!*

Q   I'm useless at maths. What's an easy way to cut calories without having to count them?

A   *One easy way to cut back on daily calorie intake is to employ a 'starch curfew' in the evening, after 5 p.m. That means no rice, potatoes or pasta with your evening meal, and no bread. Instead, you can have a feast of a portion of lean protein (about the size of a deck of cards) such as fish, chicken or tofu, and a massive leafy salad, or a plateful of steamed vegetables. If you want a pudding, then base it on fruit (cakes, biscuits and pastries count as starch). You'll cut back on around 300–400 calories and, as you're doing it in the evening when most people's energy requirements start to wind down, you shouldn't feel deprived. Do this every day without making any other changes and you should lose half a kilo of fat every eleven days.*

18
Supplementary benefits

Most nutritionists believe everyone will benefit from taking a good multivitamin and mineral supplement every day.

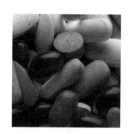

But what else should you take if your goal is living younger for longer?

How many times have you read that a healthy, balanced diet should provide all the vitamins and minerals a body needs, and that supplements are a waste of money? In theory, it sounds reasonable. But it doesn't explain why virtually every anti-ageing researcher and scientist takes supplements on a regular basis.

Let's face it, we never quite live up to our healthy intentions. We know we need five portions of fruit and vegetables a day, but average consumption is just about half that. On top of this certain lifestyle factors, such as smoking and heavy drinking, can deplete your body of nutrients, and stress can also take its toll on the B vitamins which are required to keep the nervous system healthy. Plus, as we age, we require fewer calories on a daily basis, and so our chances of getting the right amount of nutrients from food are reduced. Add to that the fact that modern farming and food processing techniques have reduced the vitamin and mineral content of many foods, and you can see the problem.

Here's an idea for you... **When's the ideal time to take vitamin supplements? Nutritionists say it doesn't matter, as long as they're taken at roughly the same time every day. This is to ensure that levels of nutrients are consistently topped up. You're also most likely to remember to take them if it's become part of a daily routine. Many people find the easiest way to remember is to take their supplements with breakfast, as it's the meal most regularly eaten at home. Keep your bottles next to the kettle as a reminder!**

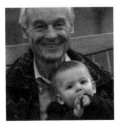

But walk into any health-food store and you can be overwhelmed by the choice of supplements on sale. It's not simply a case of 'more is better' – your body (and your bank balance) will thank you for making an informed choice of a select few. Here's a simple four-step guide to successfully negotiating the supplement maze.

1. START WITH A DAILY MULTIVITAMIN/MINERAL SUPPLEMENT

This will make up for any deficiencies caused by trace elements missing from your diet. You don't have to spend a fortune or buy it from an obscure mail order company – you can get an affordable, good quality multi from most supermarkets and high street pharmacies. Look for one that includes selenium – a mineral needed in trace amounts that's thought to boost the immune system. One study found that 100 mcg of selenium taken daily reduced the death rate among cancer patients. Ideally, it should also include around 50 mg of magnesium, which helps to lower blood pressure.

2. BOOST YOUR VITAMIN C

Vitamin C's main job is to enter your cells and lie in wait to eliminate opportunist free radicals looking to damage your DNA. When it has a spare moment, it also helps heal artery walls that have become damaged, reduce cholesterol and lower blood pressure. It's also vital for boosting the immune system and plays a big role in fighting cancer. Making sure you eat some citrus food or berries every day is essential, then add a vitamin C supplement of up to 1000 mg a day – the current recommended safe upper limit. Some anti-ageing experts recommend taking up to 3000 mg a day, although it has been known to cause diarrhoea in high doses. Try starting with two daily 500 mg doses, six hours apart.

The anti-ageing world is excited about the powers of a supplement called co-enzyme Q10. Find out why at IDEA 19, Queue up for Q10.

Try another idea...

3. BOOST YOUR VITAMIN E

Vitamin E can lower the risk of heart attack in women by as much as 40% and in men by 35%. If vitamin E is given to people who already show signs of heart disease, it can reduce the risk of heart attack by as much as 75%. In an ideal world, vitamin E likes to work with vitamin C – they complement each other as E is fat soluble, and C is water soluble, so between them, they've got the body covered. Make sure you're eating wholegrains such as wholegrain cereals, bread, rice or pasta several times a day, and green leafy vegetables at least once a day. Then add a supplement of up to 540 mg a day.

'Every human being is the author of his own health or disease.'
The Buddha

Defining idea...

4. BOOST YOUR BS

Homocysteine is an amino acid which builds up in the blood as you age. Now scientists are linking high homocysteine levels with a higher risk of heart disease. But simply taking a supplement of 400 mcg of folic acid every day is usually all you need to substantially reduce your homocysteine to safe levels. Folic acid is a B vitamin that likes to work synergistically with the other Bs, so look for a B complex supplement.

How did it go?

Q **Aren't there some supplements that can actually cause cancer?**

A *Yes – two separate studies show that taking synthetic beta-carotene may increase the risk of lung cancer and death in smokers. So avoid beta-carotene supplements if you smoke (better yet, avoid smoking and take the beta-carotene).*

Q **I've been taking them for a week and don't feel any different. Is this normal?**

A *Don't give up! No supplement is a quick fix. If you have a deficiency, you need to allow time to restore optimal levels. Many people feel better after six weeks, most after three months. In one study of top runners, a 13% improvement in performance was seen after taking the supplement for forty days. And you need to make sure you are taking it every day. If your bottle of thirty one-a-day multivitamins has lasted you all year, it's a big clue that you aren't!*

19

Queue up for Q10

Could boosting the levels of Q10 in your diet help you stave off ageing?

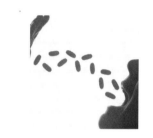

There's some compelling evidence that says it does...

It's not often that scientists get really excited, but recently there's been a lot of jumping up and down over a micronutrient called co-enzyme Q10. In fact, so much exciting research is emerging on its anti-ageing benefits, that it's beginning to look like a miracle pill. In Japan Q10 is as popular as multivitamins are; in Scandinavian countries, it's treated like gold dust – in Norway in 1994 a group of armed robbers broke into a health supplement factory and made off with 17,000 packets of the stuff, leaving the office safe behind!

Although it was discovered in 1960 (in Britain, where it was promptly ignored), it's only recently that the true extent of its anti-ageing powers has been understood. In one experiment, Q10 supplements extended the lifespan of mice by up to 45%. If humans responded like mice, this could mean an additional thirty to forty years of life.

Here's an idea for you...

Heavy drinking slows the body's production of Q10. Not sure if you're exceeding the recommended weekly limits of 14 units for women and 21 for men? Then try keeping a drink diary for a week. You may be surprised at how quickly your units add up.

So just what is this wonder substance and how exactly does it stave off ageing? Q10 is a naturally occurring substance known as a quinone, produced in small amounts by the liver and found in trace amounts in certain foods such as sardines and offal. It has two main roles in the body – it's a potent antioxidant and it's central to energy production. The problem is that it can't be made efficiently in a body that has a deficiency in any one of six vitamins and minerals, including the B vitamins (and most of us are lacking in at least one of them). Heavy drinking also affects production, and it begins to slow down altogether after the age of 40.

Some experts now believe that many of the symptoms of ageing can be linked to this slowdown in Q10 production and recommend that anyone interested in longevity take Q10 supplements. The theory is all tied up with how our cells burn food to create energy. The relevant bits of the cells are called mitochondria – the cell's energy factories. Nutrients are burned in these energy factories to produce a substance called ATP which is rather like petrol for your muscles. But, as with an engine, there are nasty by-products produced – free radicals. Co-enzyme Q10 not only helps the mitochondria produce ATP efficiently, but also helps to neutralise the destructive free radicals as they are produced. If there's a deficiency in Q10, less energy is available and more free radical damage – which ages the body from the inside – occurs. One visible side-effect of damaged mitochondria is wounds that are slow to heal.

Scientists are also getting very excited about the link between Q10 deficiency and heart disease. Q10 has been used as an experimental therapy for patients suffering from heart failure, angina and hypertension around the world. In one study involving people with congestive heart failure – a condition in which the heart becomes progressively weaker – 75% of those on Q10 survived for three years, compared to only 25% on conventional medicine. Q10 could also help your body fight gum disease, which we now know has been linked with heart disease.

Co-enzyme Q10 works as an antioxidant – your biggest ally in the war against ageing. To remind yourself of why, see IDEA 6, *Upping the anti.*

Try another idea...

Although it will be some time before there is definitive evidence of Q10's anti-ageing benefits, it also offers short-term effects that help you feel younger. It's a great energy booster and a popular (legal) pill used by athletes to increase stamina. One study even found it improved fitness levels in people who did not exercise – middle-aged Japanese women complaining of constant tiredness found that 60 mg of Q10 a day improved their fitness by over 30% – and reported being much less tired.

'Studies show that as many as 97% of the adult population is low in Q10. And if you look at the figure for heart disease, you can see the end result.'
Professor Karl Folkers, pioneering Q10 researcher

Defining idea...

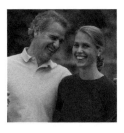 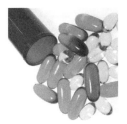

Q   I went to my health-food store for a Q10 supplement but was so overwhelmed by the choice I came away empty-handed. What should I do?

A   *You're wise to be wary – many products on sale contain too little Q10 to have any effect and it's one of those cases where you tend to get what you pay for. Q10 is not cheap, but remember the potential benefits. To get the most for your money, look for Q10 that is pre-dissolved in soy oil in dark gel capsules. Take it with food; breakfast is probably the best time as it's easy to remember to take supplements then. Athletes take 100–300 mg a day, and heart patients take up to 300 mg. For anti-ageing, take from 30–90 mg a day.*

Q   I hate taking pills. Is there any way I can get Q10 from food?

A   *It's contained in trace amounts in sardines, mackerel and offal, although you'd have to swallow pounds and pounds to reach the levels delivered by a supplement. Eating more broccoli, cabbage and Brussels sprouts can help stabilise Q10 levels in the body, however.*

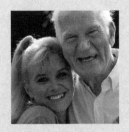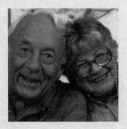

20

The right weight

If you know you're overweight but are lacking the motivation to slim, how about this? Lose weight and you'll knock years off your body age.

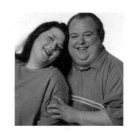

Now's the time to start, and here are some ways to help the process along.

If it's been a while since you saw your feet while standing up, you've got the food industry to thank. This extremely powerful industry spends vast amounts on advertising and marketing campaigns to get us to do one thing – eat more food. Food has never been cheaper or more readily available. When human beings evolved, we were a species that had to work hard to find enough food every day. Now, we've got to work just as hard to avoid it.

So it's no surprise that many people, men and women, adults and children, are now either overweight or obese. When you're younger, the main drawback is not looking great in jeans; you might be tempted to ignore the health risks. Once you hit 40, it's a different story. Being 13–19 kg (2–3 st) overweight at this age means you're seriously reducing your chances of being around to watch your grandchildren grow up.

I won't go on about the risks; here's just a brief summary of why it ages you. Being overweight dramatically increases your risk of cardiovascular disease, diabetes and certain cancers. In fact obesity is the second biggest cause of cancer after smoking.

Here's an idea for you...

Need an instant assessment of whether your weight is ageing you? Get a tape measure and measure your waist. It's an easy way of assessing how much fat is stored around the abdomen and whether there's enough to increase your risk of heart problems and other diseases. Standing up, measure your waist at your navel. If you're a woman, a measurement of 81 cm (32 in) or more indicates increased health risk. A measurement of 89 cm (35 in) or more indicates high risk. In men, 94 cm (37 in) or more indicates increased risk; 102 cm (40 in) or more indicates high risk.

Maintaining a healthy weight not only helps you live longer, it also improves your quality of life. People who've suffered from hormone problems, backache, joint pain and insomnia often find their symptoms disappear once they reach a healthy weight. Your energy levels will also go up, so leading a full and active life will feel natural rather than being hard work.

But losing weight is a lot harder than putting it on (don't you just know it?). Different approaches work for different people, but research has shown that people who have successfully lost weight and kept it off tend to do the following things...

IDENTIFY KEY MOTIVATIONS AND WRITE THEM DOWN

What will you gain from losing weight? Be specific, don't generalise. Do you want to suffer from less back pain or breathlessness? Do you want to be able to walk upstairs without stopping? Do you want to get into clothes you haven't worn for years? Do you want to feel better naked? Do you want to improve your self-image? Do you want to stop cringing every time you see a photo of yourself? Remind yourself of these motivations whenever you feel your resolve weaken.

THINK LONG-TERM LIFESTYLE CHANGE, NOT DIET

Read up on nutrition and learn the basics of a healthy diet. Make time to plan and shop for healthy meals. Prepare most of your food from scratch. Before you eat something, think about what nutrients it provides and what they will do for your body.

GET PROFESSIONAL HELP

Slimming clubs have a good success rate and can help to teach (or remind) you about the basics of healthy nutrition. They attract a very varied range of people, including men.

USE THE 80/20 RULE

Eat healthily 80% of the time and you'll see results. That allows you 20% for treats, such as dessert after Sunday lunch.

KEEP A FOOD DIARY, WRITING DOWN EVERY MOUTHFUL

Calories count even when the food you're eating is from your partner's plate! If you're convinced you're not overeating, write down everything you eat for a week – and that means everything, including that handful of crisps from your colleague's packet and half a fishfinger from the kids' lunch. This can be a big wake-up call.

Want to know why the longest-lived communities in the world have diets that are high in nutrients but low in calories? See IDEA 17, *Less cake, more birthdays?*

Try another idea...

'Watch your calories and stay away from greasy food.'
Angelina Strandel, USA, age 101

Defining idea...

93

Q   **I know I'm overweight but I feel perfectly healthy so do I really need to worry?**

A   We all know an overweight person who reached a ripe old age without a day's illness, but that's the exception that proves the rule. You may not have many outward signs right now, but inside it's highly likely your arteries already have fatty deposits and you may also have high blood pressure. If you are overweight and really don't want to lose it, it is possible to minimise a lot of the health risks by exercising regularly and being fit. Eating a healthy diet, not smoking, and drinking in moderation will also help. Of course, if you do all that, it's highly likely your excess weight will start to fall off!

Q   **I've got so much weight to lose it seems impossible. What's the best way to get started?**

A   Aim small – even tiny losses in weight can result in better health and lengthen your life. Lose just 5–10% of your body weight and you'll substantially reduce your risk of a whole host of diseases, from diabetes to heart disease. Losing just half a kilo a week may seem insignificant, but in a year's time that weight loss could add up to 26 kg, or nearly 4 st. So think one step at a time, slow and steady and long term. Bear in mind that research shows that the incidence of health problems due to increased weight rises almost in line with the amount of weight you put on, rather than how long you have been at a particular weight. That means your health improves as soon as the weight starts coming off – no matter how long you've been fat.

21

Get moving

The right kind of regular exercise can extend your life – but the wrong kind can shorten it.

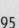

Lead an inactive life, and you increase your risk of several serious diseases. But exercise carefully, regularly, and you can slow down the ageing of the entire body.

Fact: the human body is designed to move. Regular exercise lowers blood pressure and cholesterol, produces antioxidant enzymes and cuts heart attack risk by up to two-thirds. In fact, some researchers believe that not exercising is as great a risk factor for heart disease as a twenty-a-day cigarette habit.

In fact, being fit and exercising can make up for a multitude of other sins – even smoking or eating a high-fat diet (although it's a much better idea to ditch these habits altogether). If you're fit, you're over one and a half times less at risk from premature death than someone who lives a healthy life, but who doesn't exercise.

Here's a simple way of checking your fitness level. Find your resting heart rate by taking your pulse in the morning before you get up. Press your fingers (not your thumb) on the main artery in the side of your neck, just below the jawbone. Using a watch with a second hand or a stopwatch, count the number of heartbeats in six seconds. Multiply this by ten to get your resting heart rate. Now, step up and down on a step or low bench, alternately leading legs for three minutes. Rest for thirty seconds then take your pulse for six seconds and multiply the result by ten. This is your recovery heart rate. The nearer it is to your resting heart rate, the fitter you are. If it takes more than ten minutes to return to your normal rate, your fitness level is ageing you.

And consider this: exercising will give you prompt – and noticeable – returns. Within a week of beginning a regular exercise programme, you improve your sense of well-being. Your energy levels rise and your muscles feel stronger, so every movement feels easier. The result is that you feel, and look, younger.

It's also never too late to start – studies have shown even nursing home residents in their nineties can improve their mobility by exercising. And the American Council on Exercise cites a study of five men who took part in an aerobic capacity test in 1966 when they were 20. Researchers revisited these five men in 1996. At 50, the men were an average of 25% heavier than they had been at 20, and their aerobic capacity had declined by 11%. Back on a monitored exercise programme for six months, the men increased their aerobic capacity by an average of 15% – in other words, they were more cardiovascularly fit than they had been thirty years previously.

Aerobic exercise improves your ability to process oxygen. From the lungs, oxygen travels down to the haemoglobin of the red blood cells and through the circulatory system to every cell in the body. The fitter you are, the more oxygen you can take on board and the better your body functions at a cellular level. Plus, the increase in free radicals triggered by using extra oxygen to exercise causes the body to boost production of its own antioxidant enzymes. These remain active even when the exercise stops, which means you get better protection against the oxidative stress that causes heart disease and cancer.

If you've never exercised before, you can't beat walking for a cheap, easy and effective way to start. See IDEA 22, *Walk the walk*.

Try another idea...

But moderation is the key. Forget 'no pain, no gain'. Very intense exercise can actually *increase* your risk of disease, leading to premature death, as it produces excessive amounts of free radicals that the body doesn't have a chance of mopping up. The result is a suppressed immune system that's more prone to infection and, some scientists believe, developing cancer. (If you're an athlete, don't think you're doomed to an early grave – you can minimise the effects of the free radicals you're producing with a diet high in antioxidants.)

The truth is that just half an hour of moderately intense activity can bring about the anti-ageing effect. It also has an accumulative effect so you could simply do three ten-minute sessions a day to gain the benefits. Now, what's stopping you?

'Those who think they have no time for bodily exercise will sooner or later have to find time for illness.'
Edward Stanley, US Congressman from 1837–1843

Defining idea...

How did
it go?

Q Exercise just doesn't come naturally to me – I gravitate towards lying on the sofa. Am I a hopeless case?

A *No, you're completely normal. Anthropologists have a term for this resistance to exercise – the principle of least effort. It states 'any creature, when having a task to perform, will select the way of performing the task that requires the least effort'. Today's lifestyle makes it possible to select no effort whatsoever, and the human body is not designed to be inactive. So becoming a committed exerciser can feel like you're fighting against instinct. But it can also become a habit if you stick to it three times a week. Some people never lose that feeling of dread before a run or exercise session, but they've stuck at it. Why? Because it makes them feel great – both immediately and in general.*

Q I want to start running regularly as it's such a convenient form of exercise. But every time I try, I'm out of breath after five minutes. Should I give up?

A *Don't give up, just slow down! The most common mistake new runners make is starting off too quickly. Slow your running right down to almost walking pace and you'll build up your aerobic strength. Then you'll naturally start to pick up the pace after a few weeks. Many runners start by alternating running and walking: walking for one minute, running for one minute. You can extend the running periods by a minute each week – for example in week two, run for two minutes, walk for one minute – until you're running for twenty minutes continuously. But even seasoned runners stop regularly on a long run; it's nothing to be ashamed of – you need to take a drink of water and, if you're outside, stop to admire the view!*

22

Walk the walk

Walking is the simplest way to improve your fitness level and fend off the ageing process.

It's easy to incorporate walking into everyday routines, so it's the exercise you're most likely to do consistently and stick at.

Want to add years to your life in an instant? Walk! The great thing about physical activity is that its anti-ageing effects are immediate. So no matter how unfit you've been in the past, if you start exercising now you will live a longer and healthier life. But you've got to do it consistently, and you've got to keep it up. (Don't think you can rest on past athletic laurels – no matter how fit you were once, after five years of being sedentary, you have the same fitness – and body age – as someone who's never exercised at all.) This is why walking is such a great anti-ageing exercise choice.

At this point, you're probably thinking one of two things: walking isn't real exercise, and that you do a lot of walking anyway and you're still not fit. Well, brisk walking – the pace you'd go if you were late for an important appointment – raises your heart rate to between 60–80% of its maximum, the level of activity necessary for strengthening the heart and lungs. But it does so without putting undue strain on your joints – in fact, it can help strengthen bones and stave off osteoporosis.

Here's an idea for you...

Want an easy way to keep track of your walking to make sure you're doing enough to stave off ageing? Buy a pedometer or step counter, a cheap little gadget that you wear on your waistband to count every step you take. Aim for 10,000 steps a day (roughly equivalent to five miles). Experts say that's the minimum you need to do to encourage weight loss and bring with it the many anti-ageing benefits associated with lower body fat. But that doesn't mean setting out on a daily hike – every step you take throughout the day counts, be it indoors or out, fast or slow.

Regular walking will also reduce your risk of heart disease, stroke, diabetes, high blood pressure, bowel cancer and arthritis – as well as psychological conditions such as anxiety, stress and depression. Now studies have shown that regular walking is also good for the brain and can help stave off Alzheimer's. It can also help you lose weight – one study tracked a group of walkers who did a two-mile, hilly route, three times a week. They lost an average of 6.5 kg (14 lb) in three months – without dieting.

Think you already do a lot of walking and aren't fit? You won't get results by walking the kids to school if you go at snail's pace. You should feel warm, sweaty and slightly breathless. Ideally, you should schedule some walking sessions three to five times a week, and work up to doing an hour at a time. On other days, try to fit in three ten-minute walks throughout the day.

For best results, invest in a good pair of trainers and wear comfortable clothing – it doesn't need to be sports kit. Dress in layers – for example a T-shirt, then a sweatshirt which you can take off and tie round your waist when you warm up. A lightweight running jacket is a good investment as it keeps out rain and wind without weighing you down.

Always warm up with five minutes of easy walking before picking up the pace. Then cool down with five minutes of easy walking at the end, and do some stretches. During your walk, keep your tummy muscles pulled in tight to support your back. Think 'tall' – don't slump into your hips. Relax your shoulders and let your arms swing naturally by your sides. Use your natural stride – don't try to lengthen it – and strike the ground with the heel first, rolling through the foot then pushing off with the toe.

Walking is a great way to boost bone density and stave off osteoporosis. For more see IDEA 44, *Bone up*.

Try another idea...

Complete beginners should start with short bursts of walking interspersed with rest periods. Try walking briskly for five minutes, walking slowly (or completely resting) for three, then walking briskly for five. Do this three times a week for two weeks, then start to add a minute a week to the brisk walking bursts. When you feel your fitness improve, begin cutting back on the rest periods. Your aim is to walk briskly for thirty minutes.

Still not convinced it'll get results? When one of the world's most respected anti-ageing scientists, Professor Jay Olshansky of the University of Illinois at Chicago, was asked which single product people should buy to stave off ageing, he replied 'a good pair of walking shoes'.

'How do you live a long life? Take a two-mile walk every morning before breakfast.'
Harry S Truman

Defining idea...

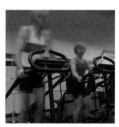

Q   I've been walking on a treadmill. Is this as good as walking outside?

A   *It's an excellent start and treadmill walking can be invaluable if it's too cold or dark to walk outside. But do try to fit in a few daytime walks outdoors every week. You'll work harder, for a start – constantly changing terrain is more challenging to the body and you have to work against wind resistance. Plus, spending time outdoors boosts your mental well-being and helps fend off depression. In the meantime, get the most out of your treadmill sessions by setting it to a hill programme to keep your muscles – and your brain – challenged.*

Q   I've been wearing a pedometer but some days I'm falling short of 10,000 steps. Any suggestions?

A   *Plenty! How about pacing around while on the phone; losing your TV remote control so you have to get up to change channels, walking all (or part) of the way to work, walking – not riding – up every escalator. (If you can't walk all the way up an escalator, stand half the way and start walking towards the top. Try to walk more steps each time.) How about getting your lunchtime sandwich from a shop half a mile away, offering to walk your neighbour's dog on a regular basis, walking around the block after dinner in the evening or planning a long walk into every weekend?*

23

Get in the swim

Not been in the pool since you were at school? You're missing out on what could be the perfect anti-ageing exercise.

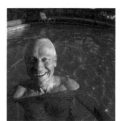

Swimming is in a league of its own. It's a cardiovascular workout that achieves the incredible feat of targeting every muscle in your body while putting virtually no pressure on your joints.

Exercising in water is like a good relationship – it's completely supportive but it also works you hard enough so that you grow stronger. You may not think so, but swimming is the ideal exercise for anyone who feels self-conscious about their body. OK, the dash from changing room to pool isn't much fun (tip: wear a towel and leave it by the side of the pool) but once you've submerged, it's impossible for anyone to scrutinize the size of your thighs, something you could never say about a multi-mirrored gym. Done in a local pool, swimming is one of the cheapest – and most accessible – ways to exercise, and it doesn't depend on the weather.

Here's an idea for you... **Want to instantly improve your swimming? Buy some goggles. They're vital to help you relax in the water. If you're squinting, your neck muscles are tense and you're much more likely to hold your head out of the water which puts pressure on your back. But don't buy cheap ones – it's a false economy; they'll leave marks on your face and fog up easily so you won't wear them.**

Of course, what we're really interested in is how swimming can stave off ageing. The definitive study assessing whether regular swimmers have a biological age that's younger than their calendar age is currently under way, but recent research already suggests that regular endurance exercise such as swimming could make you on average six years younger than a couch potato.

So if it's so great, why don't more of us do it? Basically, because we're not much good at it. Throw the average adult in a swimming pool and they do a contorted breaststroke with their head half out of the water and neck in a spasm, or a frantic front crawl that involves a lot of thrashing, kicking and head turning (and inconvenience for other swimmers). Most of us still swim the way we learned when we were desperately trying not to drown during childhood lessons at the local pool.

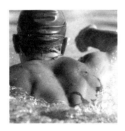
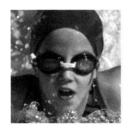

The answer? A swimming coach – cheaper than a personal trainer. A swimming coach will iron out the kinks and bad habits in your stroke until you're gliding effortlessly through the water. The newest teaching techniques draw on the body-alignment principles of the

The right breathing pattern is an essential part of successful swimming. Find out how it can also stave off ageing at IDEA 50, *Breath of life*.

Try another idea…

Alexander Technique, and the emphasis is on helping you reach a state of deep relaxation in the water. And, because your muscles are in perfect alignment, after thirty minutes of effortless powering through the pool, you will feel like you've had a massage. Done properly, swimming becomes a kind of moving meditation that you can keep up for hours.

Taking lessons is also the best way to get yourself out of a one-stroke rut. Most people find one stroke suits them best and it can be tempting just to plough up and down doing it, even if it does give you a stiff neck or tired shoulders. But alternating your strokes means you will work harder, burn off more calories and target more muscles. A coach can also design workout programmes specifically for you, using different speeds and strokes as well as equipment like floats, to get maximum results. What are you waiting for? Dive in!

'For each hour you exercise, you get roughly two extra hours of life.'
Dr Ralph Paffenbarger, epidemiologist

Defining idea…

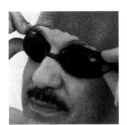

How did
it go?

Q   **I know how you breathe is important when you're swimming. But how do I know if I'm doing it right?**

A   *Most people take a huge deep breath in, then hold it when their face is under water. It's part of the anxiety many of us have about being in water – even the strong and experienced swimmers among us. To feel relaxed in the water, you should breathe normally, and never hold your breath. Try breathing out gently through the mouth when your face is in the water, then when your head comes back up, you're ready to take another breath.*

Q   **Is there anything to do in the pool except endless lengths?**

A   *How about aqua-jogging? It's as good at improving the cardiovascular system as jogging on land, and without the injury potential. It also burns around twelve calories a minute, compared with six calories a minute for breaststroke, so you can halve your time spent in the pool and burn off as much fat. All you need is an aqua-buoyancy jogging vest or belt (some pools will lend you one, or look on fitness equipment websites), and a pool deep enough so your feet don't touch the bottom. (Oh, and a certain amount of imperviousness to being stared at – at least at first.) Use the same arm movements as you would running on land. Flex and point your feet as you stride, as this will help your stability in the water. It also strengthens the muscles of the front and back of the legs. Warm up for three minutes by walking the shallow end of the pool four times. Roll your shoulders and stretch your arms above your head. Move to the deep end and do nine minutes of aqua-jogging. End with a three-minute cool down by walking in the shallow end again.*

24

Pump some iron

Lifting weights isn't just for bodybuilders.

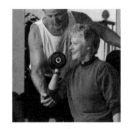

Strength training is insurance for your body — it's the single most proactive thing you can do to ensure you stay physically active right into old age.

Ever wondered at the origins of middle-age spread? Sometimes the weight creeps up because your metabolic weight has reduced. And that's happened because you've lost lean muscle tissue. Starting around the age of forty, we can lose up to a third of a pound of muscle every year. And, as muscle is metabolically active and requires more calories than fat for daily maintenance, the more muscle you lose, the more your metabolic rate declines and the more you gain weight. Even though you may not be eating a single extra calorie, this will happen.

The solution? Either cut your calorie intake or boost your metabolic rate. The only proven way to do that is to build lean muscle tissue by regular strength training. Do it regularly and you could burn an extra 300 calories a day.

Here's an idea for you... **Do open-door press-ups while you're waiting for the kettle to boil. Place your hands a little below shoulder-height on either side of an open door frame, with your legs straight out behind you, raised up on your toes. There should be a straight line from the head through to the toes. Bend your arms at the elbows so you slowly move your upper body in a straight line towards the frame, keeping your abdominal muscles held tight and your legs straight. Slowly push back to the start.**

But staving off weight gain is not the only benefit of strength training. According to a study of forty postmenopausal women, after a year of strength training twice a week for thirty minutes their bodies had become as much as fifteen to twenty years younger. All the participants *gained* bone instead of losing it as women normally do at that age, and they'd also developed muscle strength. Strong, supportive muscles and a robust skeleton mean more than good posture – they make everyday movement easier and more efficient.

The trouble is, say 'strength training' to most people and they conjure up images of dingy gyms full of large men grunting. In fact, a strength-training exercise is any exercise that puts your muscles under tension, and this can be done by using your own body weight. It doesn't have to be done in a gym, and you don't have to wear exercise gear. Grunting isn't obligatory, either!

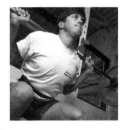
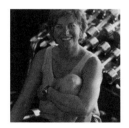

If you're a member of a gym, ask an instructor to devise a strength-training programme for you. If you want to exercise at home, here are the four top exercises to strengthen all the major muscle groups.

A youthful body is flexible as well as strong. See IDEA 25, *Flexing your options.*

Try another idea...

YOUR ANTI-AGEING WORKOUT

Aim to do this at least once a week. If you have time, do it two or three times, but be sure to leave a day's rest between sessions to allow your muscles to recover. Warm up first with five minutes of marching on the spot, and do some stretches at the end. In each case, do each exercise slowly and do as many repetitions as you can until you can't do any more (what's known as 'muscle failure'). This might be five, ten or twenty, depending on your fitness level.

1. Squats with side lift
Stand with your feet slightly more than hip-width apart. Lower your bottom as if you are about to sit down, hold for one breath then push yourself back up, raising your right leg out to the side as you do. Return to the start position, repeating the exercise and this time raising the left leg.

'Inward calm cannot be maintained unless physical strength is constantly and intelligently replenished.'
Buddhist philosophy

Defining idea...

109

2. Leg lunges

Stand with your feet slightly more than hip-width apart. Take a large step backwards with your right leg, placing the ball of your right foot on the floor. Slowly lower your right knee to the floor, bending your left leg as you do so. Go as low as you can before pushing off your right foot and returning to the start position. Repeat, stepping back with your left leg.

3. Press-ups

Start on your hands and knees, with your hands facing forward and in line with your shoulders, at a distance away from your body that equals approximately half your body width. Your knees should be behind your body and your back should be straight. Push down, taking the weight on your arms, until you almost reach the floor then push back up to the start position. Keep your abdominal muscles held tightly the whole time.

4. Front raises

You'll need a pair of dumb-bells for this exercise or two bottles of water. Stand with your legs slightly more than hip-width apart, with your knees 'soft' (i.e. not locked). Hold your weights or water bottles by the sides of your body, palms facing downwards. Slowly raise your arms in front of your body, keeping them straight, until they are at chest height. Return to the start position and repeat.

Q **Won't strength training make me look like a bodybuilder?**

How did it go?

A *No. Bodybuilders use specific techniques to achieve that look and it requires hours of focused and dedicated training. It's even harder to do if you're female and don't have lots of testosterone. Chances are, the resistance exercises described above will make you look smaller, not bigger. Pound for pound, muscle takes up less room than fat, which is why so many women who take up strength training find they drop a dress size.*

Q **I'm 60 – is it too late to start?**

A *It's never too late! In one study by strength-training guru Wayne Westcott, 85 men and women between the ages of 61 and 80 increased their muscle strength by about 50% in just eight weeks of strength training. In another study, of nursing home patients whose average age was 88, the group reduced body fat, increased muscle mass and, more importantly, saw major increases in flexibility, mobility and endurance as well as a decrease in the number of falls. In fact, the nursing home that took part in the study had to close a wing because so many residents became well enough to leave!*

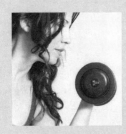 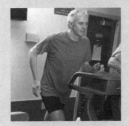

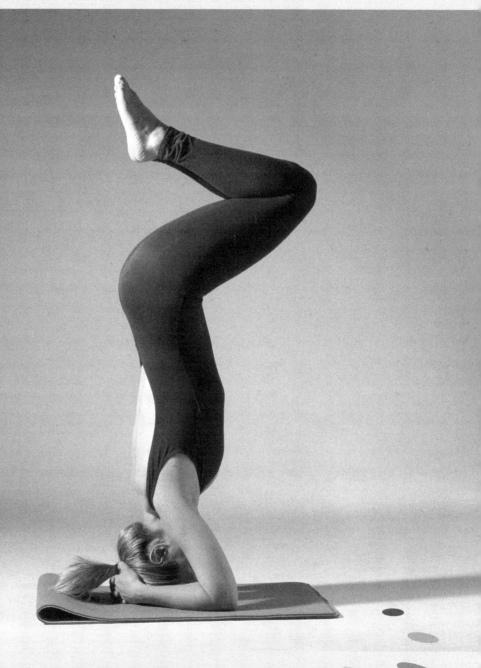

25

Flexing your options

How can contorting your body on a regular basis help stave off ageing?

Easily. In fact, if you only have time to do one exercise class a week, there are a lot of good reasons to make it yoga — especially if your goal is looking younger for longer.

Ever noticed that every yoga teacher you meet looks at least ten years younger than their real age? Or that yoga fanatic Madonna looks sleeker and fitter at forty than she did in her late twenties? It's enough to make you wonder if there's something in this yoga lark other than just being the trendiest way to exercise. And there is.

Although it's been around since 500 BC, yoga's currently enjoying a resurgence in popularity and most people now have a class local to where they live. So the chances are that you've already given it a go. In case you haven't, here's a brief summary of what's involved. Yoga is a series of postures, known as asanas, performed either individually or in a moving sequence, with much emphasis placed on specific breathing patterns throughout. Classes are usually around two hours long and end with a guided meditation.

Here's an idea for you...

Fight 'computer hunch' by doing this simple stretch at your desk several times a day to open up the shoulder area. Sit slightly forward in your chair. Link your hands behind your body, drawing the shoulder blades together. Hold for ten to thirty seconds while breathing normally.

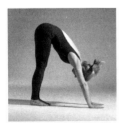

So far, so simple. But how does this help with ageing? Well, on the most basic level, the postures themselves stretch every muscle group in the body. The breathing helps as the more oxygen you take in, the more reaches your muscles and the more pliable they become. So if you can't touch your toes at the start of the class, there's a good chance you will be able to by the end. Done regularly, you'll feel more supple. Yoga can also help redress posture imbalances that, left unchecked, can lead to pain and debilitation. Take the average computer user who spends hours every day hunched over the computer keyboard. (Trust me, you hunch. We all hunch.) That can lead to the muscles in the chest shortening, and the shoulders and upper back rounding forward. And let's face it, there's nothing more ageing than a hunched back – or poor posture in general – on both an aesthetic and a practical level. A weekly class will help to stretch out the shortened muscles, but will also make you aware of your posture so you're more likely to correct it when the hunch starts to creep in.

Some yoga postures will also improve muscle strength as well as flexibility. Many use your own body weight as resistance in the same way that you would use weights in the gym. So you get increased lean muscle mass and a boost in your metabolic rate into the bargain.

Yoga is an excellent immune system booster. Find out why this is vital for long life at IDEA 4, Boost your immune system.

Try another idea...

But there's more. Yoga changes the heart rate, breathing pattern, and levels of hormones and brain chemicals. It can help fend off – or treat – headaches, asthma, hypertension, arthritis, back pain, diabetes, PMS, postnatal depression and insomnia. The theory is that as well as increasing the amount of oxygen that reaches your vital organs, yoga 'massages' your internal organs, nerves and glands, so all the systems of the body work more efficiently. The meditation component also helps to boost the immune system and lower stress levels.

Yoga means integration or wholeness – the concept of the mind and body working in harmony for optimal health. And no other exercise can offer you so many anti-ageing benefits wrapped up in a neat package.

'Your mind, once stretched by a new idea, never regains its original dimensions.'
Oliver Wendell Holmes, author

Defining idea...

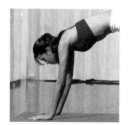 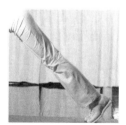

115

How did it go?

Q   It's a lot harder than it looks, isn't it?

A   *Yoga's not an easy option, especially if you've spent the last decade allergic to exercise. You've dedicated years to building up muscle imbalances so you can't expect to undo them in one session. Don't be put off by those super-flexible types who make it all look effortless. Even many yoga teachers will admit that when they started, they were as stiff as a board. No matter how inflexible you are, you will see improvements with regular practice. You'll know it's working after a few weeks when that chronic neck or back pain you've come to accept as normal starts to disappear.*

Q   There seem to be many different types of yoga these days. How do I know which will suit me?

A   *New styles of yoga class are springing up all the time. But unless they're a fusion of a different form of exercise altogether (yogaboxing, anyone?), they're all based on the same postures. There can, however, be huge differences in how these postures are presented in a class. Some teachers choose to do them in fast-paced sequences (often known as astanga). You're probably better off opting for that class once you've got a bit of experience under your belt. And talking of belts, some classes, such as iyengar, use these – and blocks – to make postures more achievable for beginners. Then there are classes which place more emphasis on breathing and meditation. There's only one way to find out what suits you, and that's by trying as many as possible, if you're lucky enough to have a choice in your area. In the end, most people find that the style of yoga is not as important as whether or not they like the teacher.*

26

The sleep solution

Don't skimp on sleep if you want to feel younger for longer.

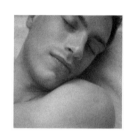

Deep sleep triggers the release of growth hormone which repairs the body's tissues.

Ever looked in the mirror after a late night and thought you looked older? It's not your imagination. When you don't get enough sleep, you miss out on growth hormone, an amazing chemical that fights the ageing process.

When you enter the deepest stage of sleep, growth hormone is released from the pituitary gland located just below the brain. It increases the amount of nutrients taken up by the cells, and increases the rate at which they divide, encouraging the growth and repair of muscle and bone, and stimulating the immune system. If you cut back on sleep, you're cutting back on growth hormone and giving your body less chance to repair itself.

The ideal amount is between six and eight hours. Get less than this and you start to build up a sleep debt and that's bad news for living longer. One study of over 70,000 nurses found that women who got five hours of sleep or less nightly over a decade had a 39% greater risk of heart attack than those who managed eight hours. It has also been found that building up a sleep debt over a matter of days can impair metabolism and disrupt hormone levels, preventing the body from processing glucose in the blood.

Here's an idea for you... **Not sure exactly how much sleep you need? Here's an easy way to find out. Set your alarm for when you need to get up, then count back six to eight hours, depending on how much sleep you feel you need. Try to go to bed at this time every night, and get up at the same time – even at weekends. If you still feel tired during the day, push your bedtime back by fifteen minutes a week until you wake up feeling refreshed.**

But it's not just growth hormone doing wonders while you sleep. Recently scientists discovered that melatonin, the so-called 'dark hormone' that triggers sleep, is a potent antioxidant fighting the ageing effects of free radicals. It's thought to be as effective as vitamins C and E as it gets right inside your body's cells where it guards against DNA damage. That's the good news. The bad news is that melatonin production seems to slow with age. To boost levels to the maximum, make sure you sleep in a pitch-black room as exposure to light blocks melatonin synthesis. Oh, and drink your morning urine (really) – it's an ancient Indian health tonic as urine contains high levels of melatonin. Not keen on that idea? Why ever not? Thankfully, there is an alternative. 'Night-time milk', now available from good supermarkets, is produced from cows with naturally high levels of melatonin. A warm glass before bed will help you sleep and boost antioxidant levels at the same time.

Very many people say they are regularly affected by sleeplessness. It's no surprise really, because we tend to take sleep for granted – and just expect it to happen. But what we do through the day has a direct effect on how we sleep at night. It's not enough just to pass on that double espresso after dinner. Ideally, you need to avoid caffeine (in coffee, black tea, hot chocolate and fizzy drinks) from lunchtime onwards. Caffeine activates the 'wakefulness' centres in the brain and can remain in the body for hours. If sleep is a problem try to restrict alcohol intake to one or two small glasses of wine early in the evening – more than this will reduce the quality of your sleep. Avoid eating a large meal later than three hours before you intend to go to bed – eating energises you by increasing your metabolic rate.

Regular exercise can help you sleep better. For more reasons to get active, see IDEA 21, *Get moving.*

Try another idea...

Try having a warm bath before bed. Studies have shown that a drop in body temperature triggers the brain's sleep response. Having a warm bath artificially raises the body's temperature, so when you cool down again, you should feel sleepy. Keep your bedroom cool. Research has shown that 16°C (62°F) is generally conducive to restful sleep, while temperatures above 24°C (71°F) are more likely to cause restlessness. Light and darkness can have a big effect on your ability to sleep and many people find their routine is disrupted when the clocks go back. Try wearing a mask when you go to bed in summer and exposing yourself to bright light as soon as you wake up to trigger the brain's 'wakefulness' centres. Cut out noise from traffic or snoring by wearing earplugs. And finally, buy the biggest bed you can afford and replace the mattress after ten years of use.

'I love sleep. My life has the tendency to fall apart when I'm awake, you know?'
Ernest Hemingway

Defining idea...

How did it go?

Q   Is it true you need less sleep as you get older?

A   *It's true that a lot of people find it harder to sleep at night as they get older. But this may not be inevitable but merely a side-effect of years of accumulated poor sleep habits. Are you exercising less and eating more? Are you drinking more alcohol or do you have more to worry about? Do you nod off while watching TV in the early evening? Cutting out daytime naps, and getting into a regular bedtime routine and sticking to it can help.*

Q   When I've got lots on my mind, my sleep is always affected. What can I do?

A   *Try setting aside thirty minutes in the evening for dealing with your worries. Write them down and perhaps think of any action you can take the next day to resolve them. Then, put the journal or piece of paper aside before bed. Always avoid stimulating activities before bed – that includes watching TV or reading a gripping book. Try 'pottering' instead, tidying and getting things ready for the next day. If you still feel anxious, try a simple fifteen- to twenty-minute relaxation exercise before bed. Sit comfortably with your eyes closed, breathing naturally. Concentrate on your breathing and try to let go of any thoughts that come into your head.*

27

Get de-stressed

A little bit of stress is good for you, but...

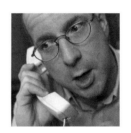

Stress is also one of the biggest causes of rapid ageing because it floods the body with free radicals. It's time to get off the stress bandwagon for good.

Stress gives you a shot of adrenaline that can be the extra kick you need to be brilliant in a meeting at work, or to swerve out of danger on the motorway. But flooding your body with adrenaline – and its side-kick cortisone – on a regular basis is also one of the easiest ways to accelerate the ageing process.

Ever wondered why you say 'calm down, you'll have a heart attack' to an overstressed colleague? Because stress hormones lead to an increase in blood sugars and lipids which increase blood pressure, a major risk factor for heart disease. It's also dangerous because it suppresses the immune system, making you more susceptible to infectious – and serious – disease. One study of healthcare workers found that those with the most stressful jobs had a lower level of antibody production than those in less stressful positions. And ever noticed that you're far more likely to forget where you've put your keys, or that you have an important appointment, when you're under stress? Stress hormones activate an enzyme in the

Here's an idea for you...

If you're worked up before you even leave the house, you're doomed. Every irritation you meet will nudge you further into the exploding zone. But start the day in a state of deep relaxation, and you may even find you don't care when you choose the slowest ticket window queue. Try some meditation. The relaxation response is an easy technique that's been proven to reduce blood pressure, breathing and heart rates. Pick a focus word with peaceful connotations, such as 'calm', 'relax' or 'love'. Sit somewhere quiet. Close your eyes and slowly relax your muscles. Breathe slowly and naturally. Each time you breathe out, repeat your focus word silently. Be passive. When other thoughts come into your mind, dismiss them and keep repeating your focus word. Aim to do this for fifteen minutes every day.

brain which affects your short-term memory. Now chronic stress has even been linked with the onset of Alzheimer's.

You know that stomach-churning feeling you get when the pressure's on? Stress also has a direct effect on the digestive system – not only does it cause a sharp fall in gastrointestinal secretions, but the body also directs blood away from the digestive system to the heart and lungs to allow you to run away from danger. So as well as being more prone to stomach upsets, your body doesn't get a chance to absorb the nutrients in food properly.

Sure signs that you're suffering from stress include being irritable and short-tempered, and having no sense of humour. Obviously, this may simply be your real personality, but it's more likely to be stress if you're also prone to headaches and stomach upsets, getting more colds than normal, bursting into tears easily, sleeping badly, drinking too much, eating more than usual or losing your appetite.

When we think of stress, we tend to conjure up major life events such as divorce, redundancy or moving house. But stress is more likely to be ongoing and low level in the form of the minor irritations that we face on a daily basis. A late train, a flat tyre, a long queue, an irate client on the end of the phone.

One of the most effective ways of combating stress is exercising regularly. Find more reasons to do this at IDEA 21, *Get moving*.

Try another idea...

Stress can be a message from your body that you need to make some life changes, like take better care of yourself, get more support or work smarter and not harder. But not always. Sometimes it's just a message that you need to change your mindset. You have little control over the daily irritations you face, but you do have complete control over how you react to them. The key is stepping back from a situation and realising when it's out of your control, then not allowing yourself to get worked up about it. You could even take it one step further and find something positive you could take from the situation. Your train's late again, but it gives you more time to read that page-turning bestseller you're in the middle of...

Remember as Charles Peirce, the founder of the pragmatic philosophy movement, said: 'The greatest weapon against stress is our ability to choose one thought over another.'

'Don't sweat the small stuff. And it's all small stuff.'
Richard Carlson, author

Defining idea...

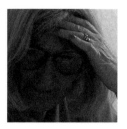
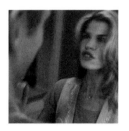

How did
it go?

Q **It's no good, my journey to work is still winding me up. Except now it's worse because I'm worrying about the effect it's having on my health! How can I calm down?**

A *Buy an iPod and download hours of the most soothing music you can find (think Handel's* Water Music *or* Spring *from Vivaldi's* Four Seasons*). People who delivered impromptu speeches while listening to relaxing classical music showed no jump in heart rate, blood pressure or the stress hormone cortisone. Those who made a speech in silence turned into stress monsters. So there's a lot to be said for the power of music, and tuning in and tuning out on the way to work.*

Q **It's my work colleagues that really wind me up. Other than locking my office door, what can I do when they bother me?**

A *Count to eight. Exhale fully and place your tongue on the roof of your mouth, behind your front teeth. Inhale through your nose for a count of four. Hold your breath for seven counts if you can and exhale with a loud whooshing sound through your mouth for eight counts. Repeat for two minutes. Result? You'll feel great and your colleagues will give you a wide berth.*

28

The sex factor

People who have frequent sex live longer than those who don't.

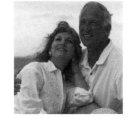

We've known for a long time that a good relationship helps you live longer. Here's how to put the passion back into your life.

Men who are happily married live six years longer than single men. They're also far less likely to develop cardiovascular disease than unmarried men, even if their cholesterol levels are much higher. Women live around three years longer if they're married.

But it's not just marriage that's good for you. Now we know that a healthy sex life can keep you young. One study of 3500 people who looked on average ten years younger than their real age found that most were making love around three times a week (the average is around once a week). In fact, if you're a man and you have sex more than average, that is twice a week or more, you're far less likely to die from all causes than those men having sex once a week or less.

Here's an idea for you...

If your image of the typical sex-shop customer is a dodgy looking bloke in a grubby mac, you've obviously never been to one of the new ones springing up all over the place. They're full of great ideas for great nights in with your other half. Many are open in the evenings so why not visit one together on your next night out? If you really can't face it, or there isn't one near you, many of them have websites. Check out www.coco-de-mer.co.uk, for instance.

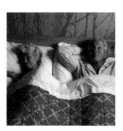

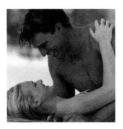

Not only is sex thought to be good exercise, improving cholesterol levels, increasing circulation and releasing endorphins, it may also release chemicals that benefit the immune system. Frequent ejaculations in men may reduce the risk of prostate cancer by as much as 33%.

It seems straightforward enough – have more sex if you want to live longer. Except that it's not just something you can simply add to the bottom of your daily 'to do' list ('ring accountant, sort out the shed, defrost supper, have sex'). If you've been in a relationship for several years you may be well past the 'ripping each other's clothes off' stage. Your body may be feeling the effects of both gravity and a bit of extra weight. That's normal and of course it doesn't mean you're no longer attractive. But it's easy to feel like that when you're surrounded by air-brushed images of nubile, scantily-clad sex goddesses (and gods) in the media, even if you do remember that the pictures are often doctored to make them look that good. So having sex more often is not just going to happen – you have to make it a bit of a project.

Platonic friendships are also vital to a long and healthy life. Find out how at IDEA 32, *Mingle!*

Try another idea...

One of the main reasons we go off sex with our long-term partners is because there are so many distractions in life – paying the bills, doing the washing up, dealing with each other's families and the kids. Sex arises out of the quality of a relationship as a whole. To prioritise your sex life, you have to strengthen the whole relationship, of which sex is just a part. So forget the dishes, leave the answerphone on and sit down to pay each other some real attention. Make time to have a glass of wine and a chat together. Don't just talk practicalities, talk about your hopes and dreams. And make each other laugh!

Then put a little imagination into trying something new. It doesn't need to be superkinky – something as simple as scented massage oil and candlelight can work wonders. Experimenting is the best way of finding out what works for both of you. Now, when has homework ever been as much fun?

'Remember, if you smoke after sex, you're doing it too fast.'
Woody Allen

Defining idea...

127

How did it go?

Q   Do old people really have sex?

A   *Yes, of course they do, lots of it, everywhere. Although if you believe the images we're fed by the media, the only people who ever have sex are under 25 and stunningly good-looking. But many couples find their sex life improves with age. A recent report found that 44% of the over-65s who were surveyed spent more than two hours a week making love. Another – of married and single men and women over 65 – found that most people described sex as being vital to their quality of life. Older women reported that one of the major reasons they believed sex became more pleasurable as they got older was because they no longer had to worry about contraception. Sex was also seen as a means of easing tension within marriage and as a wonderful tool for diffusing arguments, improving self-esteem, emotional well-being and body image. Pretty much the same as it is for younger couples, then.*

Q   My husband finds it a bit harder to perform these days. Should we try Viagra?

A   *Some sexual slowing-down with age is natural and most men take longer to become aroused. It's a long way from impotence, but it can cause panic. Your husband may fear that he's going into a speedy sexual decline and will soon be unable to perform at all. In fact, some health conditions, such as diabetes or high blood pressure, can interfere with sexuality. It's usually temporary but there is a danger that 'performance anxiety' will take over, so the fear becomes a self-fulfilling prophecy. So above all, try to relax, and accept the changes. And don't try Viagra without first speaking to your doctor.*

29

Game for a laugh

Laugh up to fifteen times a day and live up to eight years longer. True!

Laughter reduces stress, lowers blood pressure, relieves pain, oxygenates the blood and strengthens the immune system. So go on, have a chuckle.

Two hunters are out in the woods when one of them collapses. He doesn't seem to be breathing and his eyes are glazed. The other guy whips out his phone and calls the emergency services. He gasps, 'My friend is dead! What can I do?' The operator says, 'Calm down, I can help. First, let's make sure he's dead.' There is a silence, then a shot is heard. Back on the phone, the guy says, 'OK, operator, now what?'

That is officially the world's funniest joke – and if you laughed when you read it, you've given your immune system a huge boost. It seems laughter really is the best medicine and there's a raft of scientific studies to prove it.

If you've ever been stuck in a lift when someone's made a funny remark, you'll know that nothing relieves tension like laughing. Both physically and psychologically, laughter acts as a safety valve for the discharge of nervous tension.

Smile more and you'll feel happier. Studies on brain activity have shown that if you move your face into a smile, happy-chemicals are automatically released from your brain. So smiling more has the end result of, well, making you feel like smiling more. And it takes half as many muscles to smile as it does to frown.

Researchers have shown that laugher reduces the levels of the stress hormones cortisone and adrenaline and boosts the number of infection-fighting white T-cells in the body. During laughter, the heartbeat quickens and blood pressure rises; after laughter, both heart rate and blood pressure drop to a point that is lower than its initial resting rate. It's also thought that laughter may have evolved as a way of helping us to connect with fellow human beings and dissipating conflict. As comedian Alan Alda put it, 'When people are laughing, they're generally not killing one another'.

Doctors are now realising just how important laughter is to our health and are beginning to take jokes, er, seriously. In the 1960s, the award-winning writer Norman Cousins put his full recovery from a usually irreversible and crippling connective tissue disease down to a regimen that – among other therapies – included laughing at Marx Brothers movies every day. The book about his experience was an international bestseller.

'Laughter is a tranquilliser with no side-effects.'
Arnold H Glasgow, psychologist

Laughter may even improve your physical fitness. Have a real belly laugh and around 400 muscles of your body will move – it's like internal aerobics. It releases the same endorphins or pleasure chemicals in the brain as exercise, which induce feelings of well-being and relaxation. If you could keep up a belly laugh for a full hour, you could even laugh off as many as 500 calories.

Laughter's a great way to reduce your blood pressure. For more ways, see IDEA 41, *Under pressure*.

Try another idea...

The problem is that the older we get, the more it takes to make us laugh. At 4 we laugh 400 times a day. By age 30, it's down to around 15. A small child doesn't need searing political satire to raise a smile. They'll laugh at any noise that vaguely resembles passing wind. Or just get three of them together, wait until one of them says 'wee-wee', then watch them all lie on their backs and laugh hysterically for ten minutes. When did we lose this sense of fun?

Deciding to laugh more every day sounds like a simple way to live longer, but it's easier said than done. You can't force laughter. But you can polish up a rusty sense of humour by using it more often. If you've got in the habit of watching 24-hour news channels, get some DVDs of comedy films or a collection of Simpsons videos. Swap jokes by email. Hang out with some small kids.

To get you started, here's a joke.
Sherlock Holmes and Dr Watson are going camping. They pitch their tent under the stars and go to sleep. Sometime in the middle of the night Holmes wakes Watson up. 'Watson, look up at the stars, and tell me what you deduce.' Watson says, 'I see millions of stars and even if a few of those have planets, it's quite likely there are some planets like Earth, and if there are a few planets like Earth out there, there might also be life.' Holmes replies 'Watson, you idiot, someone stole our tent!'

'One laugh is worth two tablets.'
Freddie Frankl, psychiatrist

Defining idea...

How did it go?

Q   **I tried saying 'wee-wee' at work yesterday but no one laughed. Why is this?**

A   *As every comedian will tell you, it's all in the timing. There's even a joke about it. A man goes to a prison and everyone is having lunch. Someone shouts out 'Twenty-three', and everyone falls about laughing. The man asks what's going on. Someone tells him. 'Because we've heard all the jokes we've numbered them all. Here, listen. Forty-eight!' It gets a big laugh. 'Let me try,' says the man. 'What's a good one?' 'Sixteen,' replies the inmate. The man shouts 'Sixteen!' There's no response. The other inmate leans over. 'It's not just the joke,' he says, 'it's the way you tell them.'*

Q   **Sometimes if I really laugh I start to cry. Is this normal?**

A   *Normal and pretty common – if the saying 'crying with laughter' is any indication. It's thought to be all tied up with stress release – having a good cry can be as big a tension reliever as a belly laugh. It just tends not to go down so well at the office.*

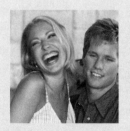
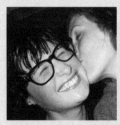
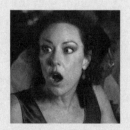

30

Sweet success

You don't have to be rich to live a long and healthy life. But you do need to be socially successful. And maybe win an Oscar...

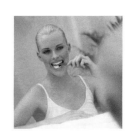

We can learn a lot about longevity from Oscar winners. It seems that the more successful you are, the longer you live.

They've got living longer sussed. On average, Oscar winners live four years longer than non-Oscar-winning actors, and actors winning many Academy Awards live an average of six years longer.

It's not just actors. How educated you are also makes a difference, with PhDs living longer than those with master's degrees, and those holding master's degrees living longer than those with Bachelors of Arts. Managers live longer than clerks, but not as long as chief executives. But it's not simply because the more successful among us have access to the best healthcare, not to mention nutritionists and personal trainers (although that does help).

Here's an idea for you...

You'll live longer if you feel like a success. But it's up to you how you define success. It could mean turning down a well-paid job to do something you find more fulfilling. It could be feeling fitter, stronger and more vital with every year. Or it could be as simple as being honest and authentic in your dealings with other people at all times. Take a few moments to think about what success means to you and write down a short description. It's always easier to work towards a goal that's clearly defined.

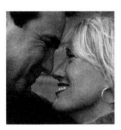

Defining idea...

'Live long and prosper.'
Mr Spock, *Star Trek*

It all comes down to your position in the social hierarchy, according to Professor Michael Marmot, the world-renowned epidemiologist who came up with the theory after thirty years of research. If you want to live a long life, you need to scramble to the top of your particular social pile. He found that between the ages of 40 and 64, you're four times more likely to die if you're at the bottom of the pile than the top.

How much money you have is unimportant – provided you have more than those around you. It's so important, that most of us would actually take an income cut if it could guarantee we'd still be earning more than anyone else. (In one study, a group of students were offered two options. Earn $125,000 a year, in a society where everyone else earns $100,000 a year, or earn $175,000 with everyone else earning $200,000. They all opted to earn the lesser amount of $125,000, but being richer than their peers.) Even small moves up the hierarchy, such as a promotion at work or moving from a three- to a four-bedroom house, can lead to a longer life.

Being seen as a success and held in esteem by your peer group has a powerful effect on the immune system. It's also boosted by feeling that you're in control of your life. You may

To find out more on how a good social life can help you live longer, see IDEA 32, Mingle!

Try another idea...

work eighteen-hour days when you're the boss but your stress levels may well be lower than the lowliest employee who has a mundane job. Why? Because one of the greatest causes of stress is lack of control over your own life. And we already know that high stress levels lead to increased rates of heart disease, stroke and even cancer.

It's also crucial to feel in control of your working life, so ask yourself some key questions. What aspects of my job are beyond my control? Is there anything I can do to change the situation? If not, can I change how I react to the situation? What aspect of my job empowers me? Can I do more of it? Do I need to work for a different boss? Do I need a different job?

If you're stuck in a dead-end job, or just allergic to hard work and ambition, you're not doomed. Concentrate on being popular instead. It's thought that being held in high esteem by your close friends and family, and having plenty of opportunities to get out and meet people, can counteract the negative, ageing effects of a menial job.

'Success is liking yourself, liking what you do, and liking how you do it.'
Maya Angelou

Defining idea...

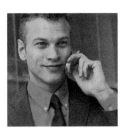

135

How did it go?

Q   **I've joined an amateur dramatics group. Now, how do I get nominated for an Oscar?**

A   *You can experience the effects of winning an Oscar without setting foot in Hollywood, according to the scientists behind the theory. They believe that winning an Academy Award gives you an inner sense of peace and accomplishment that can last for your entire life, which alters the way your body copes with stress on a day-to-day basis. But any sense of achievement will have the same effect. So simply landing a role in your next amateur production and doing it well could help you live longer. And psychologists believe that starting and finishing even minor tasks like weeding the garden or painting a room can improve your mental health. Apparently, when you get close to accomplishing something, your brain sends out 'reward' signals that lift your mood and boost your immune system. So the message is don't just sit there, do something!*

Q   **I've got into a bit of a rut over the years and now the thought of change makes me anxious. What can I do about it?**

A   *Remember, if you do what you always do, you'll get what you've always got. If your goal is to feel more youthful, vital and energetic, you need to make changes and this can be frightening. But the irony is that those who never take any risks live with a dread of something going wrong. They seek security above all else, but the effect is chronic insecurity. It is actually easier (and infinitely more life-fulfilling) to try new things. The decision to incorporate more challenge into your life will ultimately bring a feeling of security because you'll know you can tackle anything. So choose a small step, and take a big leap. You'll be amazed at how good it can make you feel.*

31
Let the spirit move you

You've got to have faith. If you want to live longer, that is.

Be a good person and you won't have to wait for the next life to reap your rewards. You'll live a healthier life for longer in this dimension — on average, seven years longer.

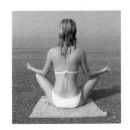

Study after study has shown that people who worship regularly live longer than those who don't. They tend to have lower blood pressure, lower death rates from cardiovascular disease, less depression and less early death from various causes.

Scientists, being practical people at heart, are confounded by the idea that sitting in a chilly stone building and singing along to some organ music once a week can have such an effect on health. They've tried to explain it away by saying that worshippers tend to have healthier lifestyles, such as not smoking, exercising regularly, keeping up social contacts and staying married, and it's these choices that keep them full of life for longer. But it seems that it's not as simple as that. What scientists are discovering is that having faith, of any kind, has a powerful health-protective effect all of its own.

Here's an idea for you...

Not sure about praying? Then try counting your blessings instead – every day, write down three good things (big or small) that happened, and ask 'Why did this good thing happen?' Research shows that people who do this for a week are significantly happier three months later.

It's having a belief in a higher purpose, and taking time out to concentrate on the bigger picture on a regular basis, that gives the immune system a significant boost. Going to a church (or temple, or synagogue, or whatever) is one way of doing this, but organised religion isn't to everyone's taste. Developing a spiritual life that works for you will have the same effect.

Take prayer. You may not have said a prayer since you used to ask God to bless mum, dad and your pet rabbit. Or you may associate it with simply repeating ritualised scripts that don't make a lot of sense. But prayer is essentially a form of meditation, a time of stillness, that can do quite astonishing things for your well-being. You don't have to do it on your knees, if you don't want to. The key is setting aside some time to focus your mind.

For the past thirty years, Harvard scientist Dr Herbert Benson has conducted hundreds of studies on prayer. He focuses specifically on meditation, the Buddhist form of prayer, to understand how mind affects body. All forms of prayer, he says, evoke a relaxation response that quells stress, quiets the body, and promotes healing. Brain scans taken when someone is praying show that the limbic system which regulates relaxation, heart rate, blood pressure and metabolism is activated.

Defining idea...

'Scepticism is the beginning of faith.'
Oscar Wilde

Other scientists believe that faith or a sense of spirituality can give you a 'world view' – a perspective on problems that help you better cope with life's ups and downs. Having such a world view helps people cope with difficult life changes and relieves the stress that goes along with them.

Searching for spirituality that works for you? Some people find that yoga helps. For more good reasons to do it, see IDEA 25, Flexing your options.

Try another idea...

Psychotherapist Robert Holden puts it another way. He believes that there is a level of your mind which is all about God – whether you are religious or not. He suggests simply asking your highest Self, or God if you prefer, for some light. Then imagine a light shining in your mind. Relax and welcome the feeling it brings.

'Faith is the art of holding on to things your reason has once accepted in spite of your changing moods.'
C S Lewis

Defining idea...

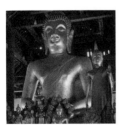
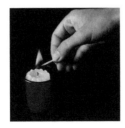
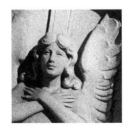

How did it go?

Q **I like the idea of praying, but I'm unsure how to start. What sort of thing should I say?**

A *There's no need to learn and repeat written prayers, or use a lot of ancient language like 'thee' and 'thou'. What's important for your well-being is giving thanks for good fortune. It's a way of reminding yourself about what's good in your life. You could then move on to your worries, hopes and dreams, and make simple requests for help. Many people find a quick prayer before sleep helps to calm anxieties that might keep them awake.*

Q **I'd love to learn to meditate but I just don't have time. What's the easiest way to do it?**

A *There are loads of simple meditation techniques to try. One of the most effective is candle gazing – sit in a quiet place and gaze at the flame of a lighted candle for five minutes. Now close your eyes and concentrate on 'gazing' at the flame image in your mind. Hold it for as long as you can. But if you're tired and stressed, you can't beat meditating on the floor. Lie flat with your palms on the floor by your sides. Lie still for a few seconds, letting your thoughts gradually quieten down. Feel the weight of your body sinking into the floor. Now, concentrate in turn on each part of your body, noticing any areas of tension and allowing the stress to melt away. Work upwards from your toes, feet, ankles, calves, knees, thighs, groin, midriff, chest, shoulders, hands, arms, to your neck and head. Then, simply lie still and concentrate on the breath, watching it come and go. Breathe in through the nose and out through the nose or mouth. If your mind wanders off in any direction, gently bring it back to an awareness of each breath you take. Let your attention focus on the sensations you can feel at the end of your nose or your lips as the air passes through on its way in and out. Relax, then slowly sit up when you feel ready.*

32

Mingle!

Want to live longer? Then join the club – literally. A strong social network can help fend off ageing.

Having lunch with a friend, visiting a relative, joining a book group or a swimming club? They've got one thing in common — they'll all help you live longer.

There's a whole body of evidence to support the idea that having a strong family network and a varied social life helps you to live longer as well as stay healthier. The immune systems of people who have lots of friendships have been shown to work better under stress than those of people who don't.

Scientists are discovering that close relationships boost immune function, help protect against disease and even speed recovery time after surgery. Studies have even shown that feeling socially isolated can be as dangerous for your health as high blood pressure, obesity, a sedentary lifestyle and possibly even smoking.

Here's an idea for you...

Boost your health in five seconds – stroke a cat or pat a dog. Time spent stroking and talking to animals increases endorphins, the feel-good chemicals in the brain, and decreases cortisone, the stress hormone that damages the immune system. If you spend a lot of time alone, it could be worth considering getting a pet – or volunteering to help look after someone else's.

What's important is having a sense of social support, and it doesn't matter whether it's from friends, family, colleagues or even strangers. Women with advanced breast cancer were assigned to two groups. All were given the same medical treatment, but one group also met once a week to talk about their feelings. Five years later, the women who were part of the support group had lived, on average, twice as long as those who weren't.

Part of the effect is what's known as peer influence – people in your social network may subtly or directly encourage you to change unhealthy lifestyle habits, such as smoking or excessive drinking. Or they may urge you to visit your doctor when you feel rough, which can prevent problems from escalating.

But social networks can also increase your sense of belonging, purpose and self-worth, promoting positive mental health. They can help you get through a divorce, a job loss or the death of a loved one. And you don't necessarily have to lean on family and friends for support to reap the benefits. Just knowing they're available can reduce the effects of stress hormones on the body. Social isolation, on the other hand, can contribute to depression and undermine your self-esteem and sense of purpose. It can also lead to feelings of helplessness and hopelessness.

Being sociable boosts your immune system, and so does having a good relationship with your other half. Find out how at IDEA 28, *The sex factor*.

Try another idea...

But boosting a flagging social life can get harder as you get older. Statistics show that more and more of us are now living alone – and in big cities, you might not even get to know your neighbours. Joining a club that interests you is a good idea as it's highly likely you'll find people there that share your interests (if they don't, why did they join the club in the first place?). It could be a hiking club, a wine appreciation class or a book group. Doing voluntary work is also worth trying – at your local hospital, youth club or museum. Or join a cause – get together with a group of people working towards something you believe in such as clearing a local waste ground of rubbish or supporting a specific charity. The possibilities are endless and it's up to you what you choose to do. Simply being involved is far more important than what you're involved in.

'Those who love deeply never grow old; they may die of old age, but they die young.'
Dorothy Canfield Fisher, writer

Defining idea...

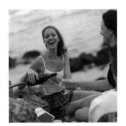
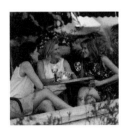
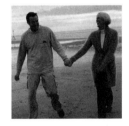

How did
it go?

Q   I'm out of contact with a lot of my old friends. What's the best way of getting back in touch?

A   *Computers have been blamed for killing the art of conversation (or was that television?) but thanks to the internet, it's never been easier to resurrect old friendships. It's a great way to trace people you've completely lost touch with. An easy first start is to 'Google' them – put their name into the search engine and see if anything comes up. At worst, you'll find out what hundreds of other people with the same name are up to! You can also sign up to specific websites designed to reunite friends from school, university and even holidays. Once you've made contact, email is invaluable. It's often easier than a phone call or face-to-face meeting with someone you haven't seen for years. It's a comfortable way to rebuild a dialogue and gives both parties a chance to decide if they want to take the friendship forward and meet up. And on a practical level, it's a good way of keeping in contact with friends who live far away.*

Q   There are some friends I've kept in touch with that I just don't have anything in common with. Frankly, they drive me mad. Are they really good for my health?

A   *As you suspect, not all social contact is good for your health. If your friends place heavy demands on your time and resources, and you feel guilty about letting them down, you'll end up feeling stressed and anxious. It's also bad news for your psychological health to feel continually obligated to other people, as though you must continually repay them for their efforts – or if you feel you must pretend to be someone you're not when you're with them. Sound familiar? Try asking a simple question: does this person empower me and leave me feeling full of hope? If they truly don't, then it's time to withdraw from them and stop making the effort to keep the friendship alive. If you do this, you'll probably end up meeting only every couple of months which you may even enjoy. Plus cutting out the energy-drainers will leave you more time to spend with friends who do make you feel good – and help you live longer.*

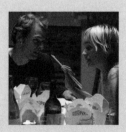
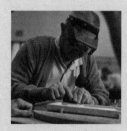
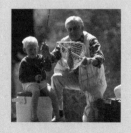

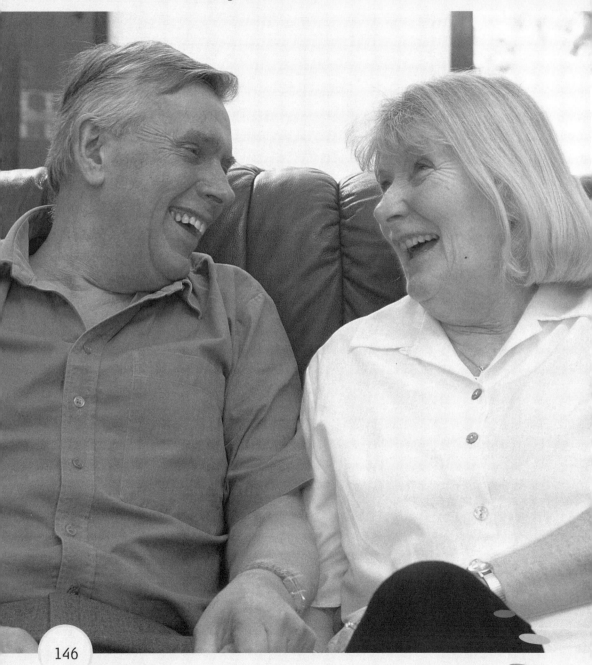

33

Mind games

Ageing is a state of mind. So can you think yourself younger?

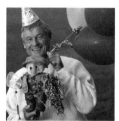

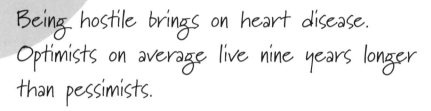
Being hostile brings on heart disease. Optimists on average live nine years longer than pessimists.

What's going on? Can you think yourself young? Does your frame of mind have a direct effect on how fast you age? You bet it does. The medical profession has only recently accepted that the mind and body are inextricably linked, but now there's a whole new branch of science dedicated to finding out exactly how the two work together. Called psychoneuroimmunology, it's still in its infancy but the one thing it can tell us is that stress levels affect the immune system.

One of the pioneers in the field is the Nobel-prize winning Dr Candace Pert, who has done a lot to prove that each cell in your body communicates with all the other cells to enable the body to work as one unit. So, changes in the brain's cellular activity caused by various emotions will have a direct impact on all the other cells in the body.

Here's an idea for you...

Perform acts of random kindness on one day a week – studies have shown it benefits you more than the person on the receiving end. Give up your seat on the bus or train for someone who looks like they need it more than you do, hold open a door, let a driver out at a busy junction, visit a housebound neighbour, smile at everyone you walk past...

The processes at work in the mind/body link are incredibly complex. Neurotransmitters in the brain can be affected by emotions and, in turn, trigger physical reactions in other parts of the body, including the systems that combat illness. And illness, of course, affects emotions and behaviour.

It's now accepted that your attitude to illness may have a direct effect on its outcome. One study suggested that women with breast cancer who have a 'fighting spirit' have a better survival rate than those who take a more fatalistic approach. Another study has shown that heart disease progressed more rapidly in men who felt helpless than in those who did not.

What else makes a healthy, youthful mindset? It's important to ditch the guilt. Research has shown that people with low levels of guilt are less likely to go to the doctor or suffer from colds or flu. It has been discovered that guilt over enjoying things like sex or eating chocolate lowers levels of immunoglobulin A, which is associated with a strong immune system.

Defining idea...

'A man is but the product of his thoughts: what he thinks, he becomes.'
Mahatma Gandhi

A youthful mental image of yourself is vital if you want to stave off ageing. Your mind is like a heat-seeking missile – it moves towards the goals you create, be they positive or negative. So if you constantly think and picture yourself as ageing, overweight and out of shape, that's what you'll be. Think of yourself as a youthful, energetic person and you'll start to act like one. Think 'I want to be someone who looks ten years younger and has enormous amounts of energy and zest for life.' Then ask yourself, what actions would this person take? What would they eat, how would they deal with stress, how would they start each day?

Laughing every day can boost your immune system. There's more to smile about at IDEA 29, Game for a laugh.

Try another idea...

If you're reading this then you're open to new ideas and enthusiastic about learning new things. That alone guarantees you'll always be biologically younger than your calendar age. Education keeps your mind active and young. You don't have to take a degree (if you don't want to). Life-long learning means keeping an active curiosity about life. Take an evening class in a skill you always wanted to learn. Try a holiday off the beaten track. Take days out to art galleries and museums. If you've got a long list of things you used to enjoy doing but no longer do – exercise, sketching, going to the theatre – it could be a sign that your mindset is ageing.

'When one door of happiness closes, another opens; but often we look so long at the closed door that we do not see the one which has been opened for us.'
Helen Keller

Defining idea...

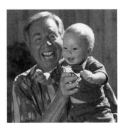
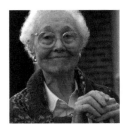

Q   **I've heard that optimists live longer than pessimists. Trouble is, I'm naturally gloomy. What can I do?**

A   *According to psychologists, optimistic people tend to interpret their troubles as transient, controllable and specific to one situation. Pessimistic people, on the other hand, believe that their troubles last forever, undermine everything they do and are completely uncontrollable. If you really are naturally gloomy – and statistics show that the number of people taking antidepressants has trebled in the past decade – psychologists believe you can actually learn to be optimistic. There's a well-documented method for building optimism that consists of recognising and disputing pessimistic thoughts. The key to disputing your own pessimistic thoughts is to first recognise them, then treat them as if they were uttered by someone else, a rival whose mission in life was to make you miserable. Visit www.authentichappiness.com for more help.*

Q   **I'm great at thinking younger. The trouble is that I never put my good lifestyle intentions into practice. What's the next step?**

A   *It takes about three weeks for a repetitive action to form new pathways in the brain and become a habit. So try making one change at a time and sticking at it for three weeks before tackling another – positive attitudes are important but don't just think! Start with something small, such as flossing your teeth or eating two extra pieces of fruit a day.*

34

Dump the Marlboro man

Why cutting out smoking is the single most important thing you can do for longer life.

You may well be tempted to skip this chapter if you're a smoker. Who needs another lecture? You need positive encouragement to help you give up — and here it is.

You know very well that smoking causes cancer and heart disease. It's written on every packet. And anyway, you're going to give up soon. Just as soon as you're over this stressful period at work...

You're probably well aware that if you're a smoker, you can expect to die seven years earlier than your non-smoking friends. The 4000 chemicals in tobacco smoke accelerate the furring-up of the arteries associated with lung cancer; with every inhalation you take in massive amounts of free radicals, which attack the DNA of your cells. One day, you may not have enough antioxidants to stave off the damage and cancer could take hold somewhere in your body. You know all this – most smokers actually *overestimate* the health risks, according to one study.

> 'To cease smoking is the easiest thing I ever did, I ought to know because I've done it a thousand times.'
> Mark Twain

Defining idea...

151

Here's an idea for you... **Put some forward planning into the next time you give up. Choose a date a few weeks in the future and put it in your diary. (Avoid 1 January whatever you do!) If you smoke at work, choose a Saturday or Sunday. If you work in a non-smoking office, you might find it easier to pick a work day. Try to anticipate tricky situations and have a plan of action in advance. Drinks after work for a colleague's birthday? Tell them you can only stay for an hour – then leave before the craving (and the alcohol) takes hold. And write a list of positive benefits of not smoking (for example, I'll find exercise much easier, I won't have to spend hours standing outside the office and people's houses in the cold and rain, I can stop feeling anxious about cancer) and read it whenever you feel your motivation wane.**

The saddest thing about this highly addictive and dangerous habit is that many smokers don't enjoy it most of the time. OK, that first cigarette in the morning, or after a meal, can taste pretty good, but after that it's never quite the same. So you light another, hoping that the next one will be better. Then the next one.

It's time for some positive pep talk and a pat on the back. Yes, you read that right. Smokers are essentially nice people with a nasty habit. It's time to stop haranguing you and treating you like public enemy number one. So here is some good news for smokers!

■ Have you tried to quit before and failed? Congratulations! You're one step closer to giving up for good. The average smoker quits ten times before finally managing it long term. So the more times you quit, the more likely you are to quit for good. Never give up giving up!

■ People manage to quit *all the time*. A lot of people are non-smokers. You could be one of them.

■ You've got a lot to look forward to. Within weeks of giving up, you'll have an improved sense of smell and taste. Now, imagine what a kick you're going to get from standing by the seashore and taking a great big breath when you've kicked the habit, and going to your favourite restaurant and really tasting how fantastic the food is…

Find out which fruit and veg contain the most antioxidants at IDEA 6, *Upping the anti.*

Try another idea…

■ The French and the Japanese smoke more than the British and Americans do, yet suffer from less heart disease and less lung cancer. This suggests that a diet high in antioxidants can help stave off the damages of smoking. Trouble is, studies have shown that smokers on average eat less fruit and vegetables than non-smokers. Maybe eating a healthy diet when you're a smoker seems like rearranging the deckchairs on the Titanic, but eating a healthy diet is more important than ever. Aim for up to ten portions of fresh fruit and vegetables a day to get your maximum antioxidant protection and give your body the best chance of staving off the ageing effects of your habit.

■ There are hundreds of people out there willing to help you give up. Don't go it alone. Ask your pharmacist about nicotine patches or gum. Try hypnotherapy and acupuncture. Ask your doctor to refer you to a smoking cessation clinic. It's a serious addiction so take a serious approach to giving up.

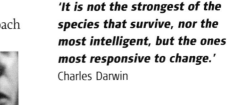

'It is not the strongest of the species that survive, nor the most intelligent, but the ones most responsive to change.'
Charles Darwin

Defining idea…

How did
it go?

Q **I used to smoke a pack a day but I gave up five years ago. How long will it take to undo the damage?**

A *Well done – and take heart. Even if you smoked well into middle age, your risk of getting lung cancer is cut by 90% within five years of stopping, Plus, it's not just your lungs that'll benefit – quitting will dramatically lower your risk of cancer of the mouth, throat, breast, cervix, stomach, bladder, kidney and pancreas.*

Q **I just can't seem to quit even though I really want to. Can I get any extra help?**

A *Yes, there's now a drug available called Zyban which can help with cravings and withdrawal symptoms. It's best taken alongside some professional stop-smoking counselling. The combination is thought to be almost twice as effective as nicotine patches. Talk to your doctor about whether or not it's appropriate for you.*

Q **I only smoke a few a day. Is that enough to affect my health?**

A *Sorry – afraid so. One in two smokers dies from their habit and the majority of these are light to moderate smokers. Heavy smokers are actually fairly rare these days. The only safe number of cigarettes is zero.*

35

Steering clear of the 'big C'

Cancer is a scary word, but more than 90% of cancers are preventable.

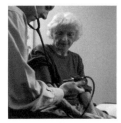

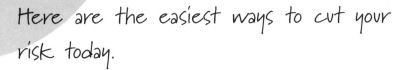

Here are the easiest ways to cut your risk today.

There's been so much publicity about medical breakthroughs in the field of genetics in recent years, you could be forgiven for thinking that cancer is something you inherit and have no control over. But you're wrong; fewer than 10% of all cancers are linked to genetic inheritance. The rest are linked to lifestyle – something we all have control over.

Let's face it, cancer is a frightening subject that gets more scary as we get older and have a closer connection to the disease – family or friends who've experienced it. But to fight your enemy you must know it so here's a simple-to-understand guide to why cancer happens – and what you can do to reduce the risk.

Cancer is a simple term for a very complex condition. It begins with just one cell that suddenly begins growing, dividing and dividing again until it forms a tumour. If it becomes large enough or spreads, it can prevent the body's organs from working efficiently which, if left unchecked, can be fatal. One theory is that this abnormal growth is triggered not by a single factor, but by a number of factors coinciding – such as environmental exposure to hazards, a reduced immune system and genetic disposition.

Here's an idea for you...

Pucker up! Did you know that wearing lipstick reduces the risk of lip cancer by 50%? It's thought to be the reason why women have seven times less incidence of lip cancer than men. Ultraviolet light is a trigger for lip cancer and by applying lipstick, whether it contains an SPF or not, you block exposure to this. And who needs an excuse to look glamorous every day? Men, don't miss out – use protective lip salve.

Most of the body (99%) is made up of cells that continually grow, divide and then die. When each cell divides, it copies its DNA into the new cell. DNA is like your body's instruction book – it contains all the information it needs to keep your body alive. Problems begin when a mistake is made in the duplication process of the DNA, or when the DNA is damaged by an attacking free radical. In both cases, a mutation occurs which is then passed on when a cell divides. It's thought that trillions of these mutations occur in the body over a lifetime but that most of them don't matter. They're either harmless or so lethal that the cell is destroyed and doesn't get a chance to divide. But there is also a very rare third class of mutations that tell the cell to begin growing and dividing uncontrollably. At this point, a strong immune system will kick into action, root out the destructive cells and remove them – which is why strengthening your immune system is your best insurance against the big C.

Unfortunately, your chances of a cancer mutation slipping through the net increase with age simply due to the law of averages – the more divisions your cells undergo, the higher the likelihood that a cancer-causing mutation will occur. But experts also believe that cancer occurs when we're older because the immune system is weakened and simply less efficient. And although it may not sound like it, that's the good news – because there's much you can do to prevent the ageing

One of the easiest ways to stave off cancer is to drink more tea. See IDEA 12, *Have a cuppa*, to find out how.

Try another idea…

of the immune system and keep it working at optimal capacity into your later years. Eating a diet high in fruit and vegetables (yes, it's that 'five a day' message again) is one of the easiest and most effective ways of doing this.

The other thing to bear in mind is that not all cancer kills. Some cancers are more harmful than others. Some cancers grow slowly, and cause little damage. The removal of a tumour, chemotherapy, radiation and other therapies can often stop cancer spreading. You could have a tumour removed in your thirties and live until your eighties.

At the risk of stating the glaringly obvious, prevention is better than cure when it comes to cancer. Your best chance of doing this is to avoid the known cancer-causing environmental factors such as smoking, obesity and poor nutrition as well as boosting the immune system so that it's better at detecting and destroying early cancers. And this can be as simple as not smoking, preventing stress, eating a healthy diet and doing some exercise on a regular basis. Now, what's scary about that?

'Since I came to the White House, I got two hearing aids, a colon operation, skin cancer, a prostate operation and I was shot. The damn thing is I've never felt better in my life.'
Ronald Reagan

Defining idea…

How did
it go?

Q   If one of my parents got cancer, does this mean I'm more likely to get it too?

A   Not necessarily. Genetics is thought to account for only 5% of cancer cases. Experts now believe that the majority of cases of cancer are lifestyle-related which means there is lots you can do to substantially reduce your risk. So try to stop worrying – nursing a parent through cancer is traumatic enough without the added stress of thinking that you're also going to get it.

Q   What's the best way of surviving cancer if you do get it?

A   Early detection is the key. If a tumour is found early, in 50% of cases, it won't recur. That's why it's vital that you keep up to date with your health checks. Women should get a smear test every three years and watch for changes in their breasts such as lumps or itchy patches. Men should check their testicles for lumps and consider asking their doctor for a prostate-specific antigen (PSA) test if they find they've been peeing more. You should both look out for changes in any moles, too.

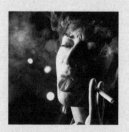

36

On the level

Some numbers are luckier than others... check your cholesterol level out.

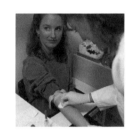

If your cholesterol is lower than 5, you'll live a longer, healthier life.

Cholesterol has had to deal with more than its fair share of bad press in recent years. The truth is, it's not all bad. In fact, we couldn't live without it. Cholesterol plays a vital role in the formation of cell walls throughout the body. It's also involved in making other essential chemicals, including some hormones.

Most of us look at a cream cake and think it's packed with cholesterol. But that's a bit of a misnomer. Most cholesterol is in fact made by the body itself. So if it's mainly made by the body, and it's essential for optimal health, then what's all the fuss about, you ask. Simple – too much cholesterol in the body is a major risk factor for heart disease, and an estimated seven out of ten people over the age of 45 have too much. And there are certain lifestyle factors that send your levels through the roof.

You can get your cholesterol measured by your doctor, and you'll be given a figure. This is where it starts to get a bit complicated. You'll be given a total cholesterol reading (ideally this should be lower than 5), but also a ratio of your LDL to HDL cholesterol (ideally, 3 to 1).

Here's an idea for you...

If you've never had your cholesterol checked, call your doctor now and make an appointment. (You can buy home-testing kits but they're not considered a good idea by most doctors; it can be hard to interpret the results.) A test involves taking a pinprick of blood from a finger. Get your doctor to write down the result for you. The numbers you are looking for are a total cholesterol of under 5 and a 'bad' or LDL level of under 3. You doctor will then take other issues into account, such as blood pressure, age and whether or not you smoke, to assess your heart disease risk.

You're probably already familiar with the terms 'good' and 'bad' cholesterol. It's connected with the special transport system that cholesterol uses to reach all the cells which need it. Cholesterol uses the blood circulation as its road system and it's carried on vehicles made up of proteins. On its journey from the liver to the cells that need it, it rides in low density lipoproteins (LDL). Any cholesterol that's not needed is returned to the liver on HDL or high density lipoproteins.

The trouble begins when there is too much LDL driving around and not enough HDL. The excess amounts of cholesterol are simply dumped on the artery walls. It's a bit like the gutters of a house in autumn when you can't clear the leaves fast enough; they inevitably get blocked with leaves and the flow of water is restricted. In the arteries, the build up of cholesterol hinders the flow of blood, which can eventually lead to a heart attack or stroke.

So your aim is to lower your LDL cholesterol (to under 3) and boost your HDL (to one or over). And one of the easiest ways to do this is to eat more fat – of the right kind. Fish oil reduces levels of LDL (bad) cholesterol and raises HDL (good) cholesterol. It doesn't have to be difficult; try a tin of sardines in tomato sauce, mashed up with a squirt of lemon juice, on a slice of toast – delicious!

Monounsaturated fats are also good news – found in high quantities in olive oil, rapeseed oil, linseed oil and linseeds, nuts and avocados, they lower bad or LDL cholesterol and raise levels of good or HDL cholesterol. Switch to olive oil for frying and dressings.

Porridge is a great breakfast choice if you're concerned about cholesterol. Find out the perfect way to make it at IDEA 15, *Porridge power.*

Try another idea...

A diet high in saturated fat (found in meat and dairy products) on the other hand *increases* LDL cholesterol and inflammation of the artery walls. In moderation, saturated fat is fine. There's nothing wrong with putting a knob of butter on vegetables, crumbling some cheese on a salad or eating a small portion of meat a day. We certainly shouldn't cut it out altogether (it's the best source of fat-soluble vitamins A and D and dairy products are good for calcium). Just make sure you eat less than 20 g a day.

Basing your diet on fresh fruit and vegetables will ensure you naturally keep fat content at moderate levels. Plus, you'll be getting enough antioxidants which help prevent LDL cholesterol accumulating on your artery walls. And finally, be as active as possible. Even moderate exercise (equivalent to walking twelve miles a week) can reduce your LDL levels.

'It is a scientific fact that your body will not absorb cholesterol if you take it from another person's plate.'
Dave Barry, US humorist

Defining idea...

161

How did it go?

Q **You can't move in the supermarket for cholesterol-lowering spreads, drinks and yogurts these days. How do they work and if I ate loads of them, would that solve the problem?**

A *The only thing you should eat loads of is fresh fruit and vegetables. But swapping these cholesterol-lowering foods for foods you would normally eat – a cholesterol-lowering spread or yogurt for your normal ones – could be a good idea. They contain sterols, compounds found naturally in plants, that reduce the absorption of cholesterol by the intestine. This frees up the liver to remove more harmful LDL cholesterol from your circulation, whilst not affecting the heart-friendly HDL cholesterol levels.*

Q **I've heard there's a drug called a statin that lowers cholesterol. Should I take it?**

A *Statins are a relatively new group of drugs which lower cholesterol by stopping its production in the liver. They've been the subject of some controversy. People who are pro-statins say that a third of all heart attacks and strokes could be prevented by using them. People who aren't so keen point out that they cause headaches, insomnia, liver problems and digestive tract problems like abdominal pain, wind, diarrhoea, and feeling and being sick. You should avoid statins if you have a history of liver problems or are a heavy drinker; first try to reduce your cholesterol levels through lifestyle changes. If this makes no difference, then see your doctor and discuss how statins may help.*

37

Get smart about your heart

Keeping your body's powerhouse young, strong and healthy is easier than you think.

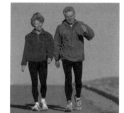

Why do so many of us have a completely fatalistic attitude towards heart disease? The truth is, heart attacks don't strike at random.

Many people believe that a heart attack is something that comes completely out of the blue, but heart disease develops slowly over several years and is more likely to produce chronic and debilitating symptoms than a sudden death. But it does kill in the end – it's the number one cause of premature death in both men and women in both the States and the UK, for example. But the truly shocking fact is that it's entirely preventable in all but a tiny minority of cases, with some simple lifestyle changes.

Heart disease, or coronary heart disease (CHD) to use the medical term, happens when the arteries leading to the heart muscle get furred up and narrowed by a fatty, porridge-like substance called atheroma. This means the heart gets less oxygen, which causes chest pain known as angina. If a blood clot forms in one of these narrowed arteries, it can stop the blood supply completely, which leads to a heart attack.

Here's an idea for you...

Your doctor (and now many large pharmacies) can check your cholesterol and blood pressure levels and give you instant results. The blood cholesterol, triglycerides, HDL and LDL are measured in units called millimols per litre of blood, usually shortened to 'mmol/litre' or 'mmol/l'. Your target is to have a total cholesterol level under 5 mmol/l, and an LDL level under 3 mmol/l. Blood pressure, meanwhile, is measured in millimetres of mercury (abbreviated to 'mmHg'). A blood pressure reading gives two numbers; target blood pressure for adults is 140/85. If you have diabetes, your target is below 130/80.

So what causes this furring-up process and how can you stop it? As you no doubt know, cholesterol is crucial. You also need to keep an eye on your blood pressure. High blood pressure – or hypertension – if left untreated for a long time, can cause the heart to become abnormally large and less efficient.

But the very first thing you need to do, if you haven't already, is give up smoking. Men who smoke more than twenty cigarettes a day increase the risk of dying from a heart attack *three-fold*. Women on the oral contraceptive pill who smoke increase their risk of heart attack by *ten* times. The reason is that many of the 4000 chemicals in tobacco smoke accelerate the furring-up process.

Exercise is also essential. It lowers cholesterol and blood pressure and makes blood less likely to clot. Just twenty minutes of brisk walking, three times a week can reduce the risk of CHD by up to 50%. Another good reason to give the car a day off, perhaps? Losing weight goes hand-in-hand with exercise – a body mass index of 25 or greater increases the risk of heart disease by nearly three times.

Cutting down on saturated fat, eating more oily fish, olive oil and loads of fruit and veg will not only help you lose weight, but will also lower cholesterol levels and stave off the free-radical damage that can affect the arteries. The

Keeping your gums healthy is another way to stave off heart disease. See IDEA 40, *Gum shield*, to find out how.

Try another idea...

incidence of heart disease is much lower in Japan and the Mediterranean countries, which is attributed to diets high in fruit and vegetables. It's thought that a regular intake of vitamin E (high in green vegetables) could slash heart disease risks by 40% in men and 50% in women. Cutting back on salt is also important as a diet high in sodium (salt) is thought to be the prime cause of high blood pressure, a major contributory factor in heart disease.

But the most recent risk factor for heart disease to be identified is an amino acid called homocysteine in the blood. Homocysteine is the opposite of your friend the antioxidant – it's a 'pro-oxidant' which can damage the walls of the blood vessels. Levels of the amino acid build up if there is a depletion of the B vitamins in the diet (and these are the commonest vitamins to be deficient – they're depleted by stress and alcohol). Taking a B-complex supplement can help reduce levels of homocysteine – and you'll probably find it really helps to boost your energy levels, too.

And now the good news. Moderate consumption (one or two units a day) of red wine is thought to protect your heart (it contains phenolic antioxidants which relax the arteries). Just make sure you don't drink more than 21 units a week if you're a man and 14 if you're a woman. Cheers!

'When the heart is at ease, the body is healthy.'
Chinese proverb

Defining idea...

Q **My father and grandfather both died of heart attacks in their fifties. I'm 47 and getting nervous – what can I do?**

A *About 1 in 500 people in the UK have inherited a high blood cholesterol level due to a condition called 'familial hyperlipidaemia' or FH. In people with FH, the way LDL cholesterol is removed from the blood circulation works only about half as effectively as normal. This means that the blood cholesterol level roughly doubles. So an adult with FH may have a cholesterol level of between 9 and 12 mmol/l, and sometimes higher. FH is almost always inherited from a parent. If someone in your family has developed heart disease early (under 55 for men and under 65 for women), get your cholesterol and blood pressure checked and talk to your doctor about reducing the risk with cholesterol-lowering drugs and diet.*

Q **I've heard that taking an aspirin a day staves off heart problems. Is this a good idea?**

A *Aspirin does seem to prevent ageing of the arteries and stop blood clots forming in damaged blood vessels. Doctors tend to prescribe 75–150 mg a day of aspirin to people who already have heart disease as it can cut the risk of heart attack by one-third. But aspirin can lead to stomach irritation, bleeding problems or an allergic reaction so don't start a daily dose without first getting the go ahead from your doctor.*

38

The sugar that's not so sweet

Staying on top of your blood sugar is vital for a longer life.

It's easier than you might think — it comes down to a few basic lifestyle changes.

Diabetes can age your body from the inside out. But the warning signs are often mistaken for tiredness or simply being run down; a lot of the symptoms can be dismissed as the side-effects of a pressured lifestyle. Others – like eyesight deterioration or going to the toilet more at night – can be seen as part of getting older. In many cases, the first time people realise they have raised blood glucose is when they go to hospital with heart problems. Many live with the condition for sixteen years before being diagnosed and treated, during which time irreversible damage may be done.

There's been much publicity about growing obesity rates and the consensus of opinion is that being overweight increases your chances of developing the disease. But don't think you're immune if your weight is normal – not all overweight people become diabetic and not all diabetics are overweight (look at Sir Steve Redgrave, Halle Berry and Sharon Stone – all have developed diabetes in the past few years). So how do you know if you're at risk, and what can you do about it?

Here's an idea for you... **A deficiency in the mineral chromium is thought to contribute to people becoming diabetic in later life. It's vital for regulating the blood sugar and insulin production but the typical Western diet is low in chromium. Make sure you're not deficient by taking a multivitamin that contains chromium, and boosting your intake by eating eggs, broccoli and potato skins.**

Diabetes is a metabolic disorder where the body becomes unable to use carbohydrates (glucose) for energy. Glucose is an essential fuel for the brain and muscles. But before it can be used, your body needs the hormone insulin, produced by cells in the pancreas, to unlock the entry gates of the trillions of cells in your body (receptors) and let the glucose in. If there's not enough insulin to do this job, two things happen: your cells don't get enough glucose to function properly, and there's too much glucose left circulating in the bloodstream. Over time, this damages the kidneys, nerves, eyesight, immune system and the arteries – diabetics are at more risk of both heart attack and stroke than non-diabetics.

But not all forms of diabetes are alike. Type 1, or insulin-dependent diabetes, usually starts between early childhood and the age of 35. It happens when the pancreas stops producing insulin altogether, usually because the body's immune system has attacked and killed 85% or more of the pancreas' insulin-producing cells.

Defining idea... **'Life is not over because you have diabetes. Make the most of what you have, be grateful.'**
Dale Evans Rogers, country singer and diabetic

Around 25% of diabetics have Type 1. The rest have Type 2, or non-insulin-dependent diabetes. In Type 2, the body is still producing insulin, but it's either not enough or not released quickly enough after eating to process all the glucose. Often, enough insulin is released but the cells' insulin receptors don't react to it in the normal way, a condition known as insulin resistance.

Red wine contains flavonoids which may counter the effects of diabetes. See IDEA 13, *The good news about booze.*

Try another idea...

You're most likely to develop Type 2 diabetes if you're overweight, as overweight people need to produce proportionately more insulin to manage their blood glucose, and extra body fat leads to increased insulin resistance. Other risk factors are being over 40, having a family member with the disease or being of Afro-Caribbean or South East Asian descent.

One of the biggest dangers of untreated diabetes is heart disease. Besides controlling blood sugar, insulin's other function is to help store fat. If there's not enough insulin to do this, or the cells are insulin resistant, the fats remain in the bloodstream, leading to higher levels of cholesterol triglycerides, raising blood pressure and impairing the flow of blood though the arteries.

If you suspect you may have diabetes, the best thing you can do is to find out for certain. The test involves a taking pinprick of blood from your finger and can be carried out by your doctor. That way, if you are diabetic, you can begin treatment promptly. If you're not, then making a few simple lifestyle changes can prevent the disease developing.

'Diabetes is as much about controlling your lifestyle as it is about controlling your health.'
Sharon Stone, film star and diabetic

Defining idea...

Q   How do I know if I need a diabetes test?

A   *Keep a diary of your symptoms for a fortnight and look out for any of the following. Do you go to the loo more than once a night? Are you prone to thrush or cystitis, or have itchy genitals? Are you always thirsty? Do you have dry or itchy skin? Are your wounds slow to heal? Do you have blurry vision? Are you always tired? Are you losing weight for no reason? Do you get tingling or numbness in the hands and feet? If you have any of the above symptoms, see your doctor for a test. Alternatively, many pharmacies now offer free walk-in diabetes tests and you can buy a simple urine test to use at home (if it's positive, however, you must see your doctor for another test).*

Q   What's the best way of making sure I never get diabetes?

A   *Losing weight, if you need to, helps bring your blood sugar levels back to normal. Exercising increases your body's sensitivity to insulin and forces your muscles to pull extra glucose from the bloodstream for up to two hours afterwards. Reducing stress levels is important as stress hormones trigger the fight or flight response, raising your blood sugar levels to prepare you for action. You could try today's trendiest diet, the Glycaemic Index, which was initially designed to control blood sugar levels in diabetics. The bulk of the diet is made up of foods which give a slow release of energy – such as beans and pulses, wholegrain bread and pasta, bulgar wheat and brown rice – avoiding peaks and troughs in blood sugar levels. You should also avoid excessive amounts of foods high in saturated fats and sugary food like cakes and sweets.*

39

Save your skin

A little bit of sun exposure can help you live longer – but too much could kill you.

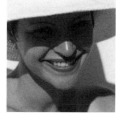

It may seem unfair, but there isn't a more effective way of speeding up the ageing process than lying on a sunlounger.

A glowing tan can cover a multitude of sins. Not only does the sun lead to wrinkles which make us look older, it also damages the chromosomes in our skin cells and can trigger skin cancer.

Ultraviolet light is the part of sunlight that damages skin. As UVB is 85% responsible for burning the skin – and has traditionally been thought to be the main cause of skin cancer – the first sunscreens mainly protected against these rays. However, around fifteen years ago scientists began to discover that UVA can also damage the skin in the longer term, by causing the release of harmful free radicals in the skin. These can suppress the immune system, cause allergic reactions such as prickly heat and damage the DNA of skin cells. The result is premature ageing – wrinkles, enlarged pores, bumps, pigmentation and saggy skin. There's also growing evidence that it is mainly UVA rays that cause melanoma – the most dangerous kind of skin cancer – and not UVB rays as was originally thought.

Never know how much sunscreen is enough? A blob the size of a large coin should cover one arm and hand or your face and neck, and two blobs will do a leg and foot, your front torso or back. Sunscreen should be applied fifteen minutes before exposure, then reapplied immediately on exposure to the sun. Reapply every two hours as it gets rubbed off. And always reapply after swimming – even if it's a water-resistant sunscreen (they're designed to protect you while in the water but no sunscreen is completely waterproof, so a certain amount will come off). Try to wait five minutes after applying lotion before lying down – a protective film forms after five minutes so it's not as easily rubbed off. You'll need one 400 ml bottle of sunscreen per person for every ten days of a beach-based holiday.

But that doesn't mean avoiding the sun altogether – the body needs to be exposed to sunlight before it can make vitamin D, essential for strengthening the immune response, healthy bones and cardiovascular health. There's also been some interesting research recently into how sunlight affects our moods, and that exposure to natural light can stave off depression. This isn't a licence to strip off and bake yourself next summer. Just ten minutes outdoors every day, without sunblock, is enough sun exposure to allow your body to make vitamin D.

Nowadays, we're clued up about the dangers of sun exposure and most of us are aware of the basic rules to protect ourselves. But what is more worrying is that the risk of sun-related cancer is determined by how much exposure you received as a child; just one incidence of sunburn as a child more than doubles your odds of getting skin cancer and DNA damage to skin can result in cancer ten to thirty years on. It's probably not what you want to hear if you're part of the generation who grew up accepting that sunburn was a part of summer. So what (if anything) can you do to undo the damage of the past and reduce your risk of skin cancer in the future?

You could start by drinking lots of green tea (around four cups a day). Studies have also shown that compounds in green tea can fight skin cancer. Stick with it – it's an acquired taste. Eating vegetables high in beta-carotene and vitamin A such as carrots is also thought to protect against skin cancers developing.

Can you buy younger-looking skin? Yes – see IDEA 51, *Looking younger*, for what products and treatments really do fight the outward signs of ageing.

Try another idea...

It's important to also keep an eye on your skin (and your partner's) – 75% of melanomas are spotted by individuals, not doctors, and with early detection almost 100% of skin cancers are curable. See your doctor immediately if an existing mole or dark patch is getting larger or a new one is growing, if a mole has a ragged outline (ordinary moles are smooth and regular) or if a mole has a mixture of different shades of brown or black (ordinary moles may be dark brown but are all one shade). You should also report the following changes if they don't disappear within two weeks: an inflamed mole or one with a reddish edge, one that starts to bleed, ooze or crust, a mole that changes sensation or one that is substantially bigger than all of your other moles.

'Nobody grows old merely by living a number of years. We grow old by deserting our ideals. Years may wrinkle the skin, but to give up enthusiasm wrinkles the soul.'
Samuel Ullman, poet

Defining idea...

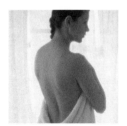
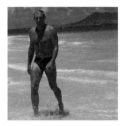

How did
it go?

Q **If I use a high-factor sunscreen, is it OK to hit the beach all day?**

A *Absolutely – as long as you spend the day in the shade. It's important to remember that sun products are not designed to extend the length of time you can stay in the sun and that UV rays can damage your skin well before it starts to burn. The biggest danger of sunscreens is that they give people a false sense of security. Many people think that they'll be safe in the sun for hours if they're wearing sunscreen – and it's reflected in the fact that sunscreen wearers are more likely to get skin cancer nowadays than non-sunscreen wearers (who are also non-sunbathers). As well as using sunscreen, you should try to avoid the sun between 11 a.m. and 3 p.m. – cover up with a hat and long-sleeved T-shirt.*

Q **Should I stick to sunbed sessions from now on?**

A *Definitely not. Although they're often advertised as such, sunbeds are not a safe option. They give a high dose of UVA light which can damage skin DNA and trigger skin cancer. One study showed that regular sunbed users were 55% more likely than non-users to develop malignant melanoma – the most dangerous kind of skin cancer.*

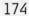

40

Gum shield

Not every anti-ageing strategy requires a major life change.

Here's one that costs virtually nothing and only takes two minutes a day.

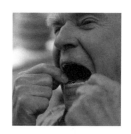

How often do you floss your teeth? It's one of those things that we all think we do more often than we do. Here's an easy way to tell – if you've had the same pack of dental floss for over a month, you don't floss enough! But there's a compelling reason to make it a daily habit: it'll help you live longer. In fact, flossing your teeth every day is such a powerful health protector it can take almost six and a half years off your real age, believes US anti-ageing guru Dr Michael Roizen.

Flossing is vital as it's the most effective way of staving off gum disease. And gum disease, left untreated, can lead to inflammation of the arteries, a major precursor to heart disease.

Gum disease starts when plaque, which is a mix of bacteria, saliva and food debris, is left for long periods on the gum surface. If it is undisturbed for around a day, the bacteria reproduce and start to become toxic, infecting the gums. These bacteria can be sucked into the lungs during breathing, where they cross into the bloodstream and are carried to various parts of the body. This triggers an immune response which causes inflammation throughout the body – including the arteries.

Here's an idea for you... **The best way to floss is to wind about 18 inches (or about half a metre) of floss around the middle fingers of each hand. Pinch it between thumbs and index fingers, leaving a 2–4 cm (1–2 in) length between them. Use your thumbs to direct it between your upper teeth; then keep a 2–4 cm (1–2 in) length of floss taut between your fingers. Use your index fingers to guide the floss between your lower teeth using a zigzag motion. Contour the floss around the side and slide it up and down against the tooth surface and under the gumline. Floss each tooth thoroughly with a fresh section of floss.**

In its first stages, gum disease is known as gingivitis. The main symptom is gums which bleed easily – you may notice blood on your toothbrush or in the rinsing water when you clean your teeth. Another major sign is bad breath that disappears when you brush your teeth, only to return shortly afterwards.

Gingivitis is easily treated with good oral hygiene; if ignored, it can lead to periodontitis or periodontal disease, where the gums recede and bacteria attack the bone supporting the teeth. Unless it's treated with antibiotics, the teeth may eventually fall out. But this is only one reason to take periodontitis very seriously – it's linked with an increased risk of stroke, and scientists have found that bacteria which grow in the mouth can be drawn into the lungs to cause respiratory diseases such as pneumonia. Severe periodontal disease can also increase blood sugar levels. In addition, gum disease is the number one cause of tooth loss for older people and it's hard to look younger than your age when you're wearing dentures.

Here are the best ways to prevent and treat gum disease.

USE AN ELECTRIC TOOTHBRUSH TWICE A DAY

Electric toothbrushes are 25% more effective than conventional brushes at removing plaque. There's also a correct technique to brushing – hold the brush at a 45-degree angle to the gumline and move the brush back and forth in short strokes. If you're not sure how to do it, ask your dental hygienist to demonstrate. Remember to change your toothbrush, or brush head, every two to three months.

FLOSS ONCE A DAY

When we brush, we tend to reach only two surfaces of the tooth – the front and back. Bacteria are then left to multiply on the surfaces between them. But 90% of gum disease is caused by the bacteria left undisturbed between the teeth. It's vital to floss at least once a day so the bacteria are dislodged and don't reach the toxic stage. If you find you're too tired to do it last thing at night, and don't have time in the morning, do it while you're watching TV or in your car in traffic jams. Most dental floss comes with instructions for use, but if you're not sure what to do with it, ask your dentist to demonstrate.

Try another idea...

Smoking may be responsible for many cases of adult gum disease. Another reason to quit – for help, see IDEA 34, *Dump the Marlboro man.*

Defining idea...

'*The first thing I do in the morning is brush my teeth and sharpen my tongue.*'
Dorothy Parker

USE A MOUTH RINSE TWICE A DAY

Antibacterial mouth rinses dislodge bacteria left behind by brushing. But don't use one which contains alcohol, as it will dry out the mouth and encourage the bacteria to breed further.

SEE A DENTAL HYGIENIST REGULARLY

You should see a dental hygienist at least every six months, or more often if you're diagnosed with gum disease. A hygienist will thoroughly remove all plaque from the gums and under the gumline – but don't worry, it should be painless.

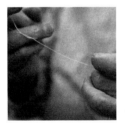 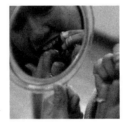

Q **Every time I floss my teeth, my gums bleed. Surely this is a sign to stop doing it?**

It's a written note in the margin: How did it go?

A *It's a sign of the exact opposite – you need to floss more often. Gums which bleed easily are showing the first signs of gum disease. But the good news is that most gum disease is curable within two to three weeks with a rigorous oral hygiene programme. You should see your dentist or hygienist as soon as possible for advice.*

Q **I'm prone to gum disease and am rigorous about oral hygiene. How come my husband, who gives his teeth a cursory brush once a day, never gets it?**

A *It may seem unfair, but women need to be extra careful about oral hygiene as hormonal changes can weaken the body's ability to fight the effect of bacteria on the gums.*

Q **Can I 'catch' gum disease from someone else's toothbrush?**

A *You certainly can. For the same reason, be careful who you kiss – the bacteria that cause gum disease can be passed on easily. Apparently, just one lip-to-lip kiss can pass on more than 500 types of bacteria, including those that cause gum disease!*

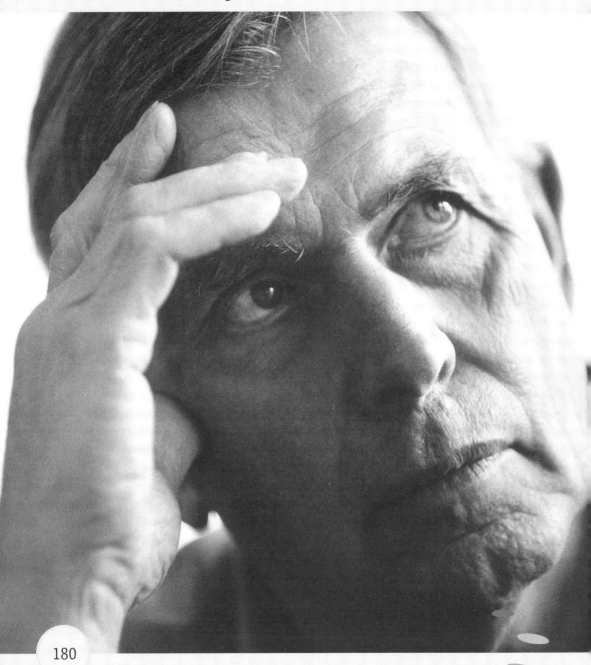

41

Under pressure

Not having a head for numbers is no excuse for ignoring your blood pressure.

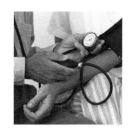

It's time to understand what the numbers mean — and how the right ones can prolong your life.

What happened last time you had your blood pressure checked? Did your doctor scribble down your reading while mumbling something like 'that seems fine'? Did you even ask what it was? Most people don't – but next time, make sure you do. And write it down.

Your blood pressure reading is always given as a fraction such as 140 over 90. And in the anti-ageing lottery, your luckiest number is 115/76. Above 140/90, you're in the danger zone – and it's estimated that around 25% of people have blood pressure above this. But hypertension, as it's known, is a silent disease, so you may have no symptoms. How does it affect how long you live?

Blood pressure is the amount of force exerted by blood on the walls of the arteries as it flows through them. The top number of the fraction refers to the 'systolic' blood pressure, which is the pressure exerted on the artery walls when the heart beats. The bottom number, the diastolic blood pressure, is the pressure exerted

Here's an idea for you...

You don't have to wear a white coat to own a blood pressure monitor. Anyone can buy one to use at home. Some use the traditional rubber cuff to take a reading, while others use a microphone to listen to the blood pulsing through the artery. Most provide a digital readout of blood pressure heart rate and will store up to ninety of your previous readings so you can track progress. They're not cheap, but it may be a worthwhile investment if you're concerned about your blood pressure (and you love gadgets).

when the heart is at rest, between beats. As you age, systolic (and sometimes diastolic) blood pressure tends to increase – mainly because the artery walls begin to get clogged up. This forces the heart to work harder to get the blood around the body. If left untreated, it can actually 'burst' an artery, and then you're in big trouble.

What's the best course of action if your blood pressure is too high? Drugs to treat high blood pressure are effective, but you have to take them every day for the rest of your life and they may have side-effects such as fatigue, depression and dizziness. And because they have no symptoms, many people with raised blood pressure forget to take their medication or don't do so properly. Fortunately, there is increasing evidence to show that lifestyle changes may be enough to bring down high blood pressure without the need for drugs.

And you don't even have to do anything weird – oh, apart from have needles stuck all over your body. There's been some interesting research recently into the effectiveness of acupuncture in treating high blood pressure and early indications are that it works and has a lasting effect. It's not fantastic

Defining idea...

'Getting old is a fascination thing. The older you get, the older you want to get.'
Keith Richards, musician

if you're scared of needles, of course. Or dislike pain (don't believe what they tell you – acupuncture can hurt).

High blood pressure, if left unchecked, can lead to stroke. Turn to IDEA 42, *Different strokes.*

Try another idea...

Eating a healthy balanced diet with at least five portions of fruit and vegetables a day and cutting right back on salt is your vital first step. Salt contains sodium and if you eat too much, your body will retain water in the bloodstream in an attempt to dilute it to safe levels. This extra volume of liquid can further increase the pressure on your arteries. Worryingly, 78% of us are still adding salt to our food during cooking or at the table – but even if you don't, the hidden levels of salt in processed food could up your intake to dangerous levels (and around 85% of our salt intake comes from processed food). We should all aim for under 6 g a day – remember that salt is often listed as sodium on food packets. (You have to multiply the amount of sodium by 2.5 to get the amount of salt in the product. So, for example, a tin of beans that claims to contain 0.8 g of sodium will actually contain 2 g of salt.)

Losing weight if you need to, exercising more and making sure you stick to the recommended weekly limits for alcohol intake will also help to take the pressure off. To really win at the numbers game, learn a relaxation technique such as yoga or meditation and do it every day.

'He who is of a calm and happy nature will hardly feel the pressure of age, but to him who is of an opposite disposition youth and age are equally a burden.'
Plato

Defining idea...

183

How did it go?

Q My blood pressure was fairly high at my last reading but I always feel a bit anxious at the doctor's. Could this have had an effect?

A   *Definitely – there's even a name for it: 'white coat hypertension'. It happens when a patient whose blood pressure is normal gives elevated readings in the surgery due to anxiety brought on by the experience itself. It's a good idea to let your doctor know if you feel nervous; it can then be taken into account. Your doctor will probably want to get you in and test regularly (you need at least three high readings over a few weeks before you're diagnosed with hypertension). Once it becomes routine, you'll probably relax more. Alternatively, ask to be tested by a nurse – many people find this less intimidating. If this doesn't work, it could be worth buying your own monitor to use at home.*

Q   Should I be more concerned about the upper or lower blood pressure figure?

A   *Both are important. In the past, the lower figure was believed to be most important. Now it's agreed that whether the top figure, or the lower figure, or both figures are high, it's important to take action. They both have an effect on your future health and how long you live.*

42

Different strokes

Why should you worry about stroke? Because it affects communication, and communication is fundamental to our lives.

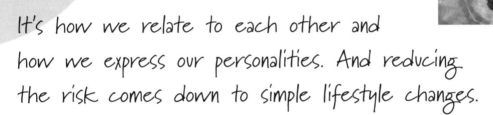

It's how we relate to each other and how we express our personalities. And reducing the risk comes down to simple lifestyle changes.

Imagine if your ability to talk was wiped out overnight. The words are in your head but you can't utter them, numbers mean nothing to you, you can't even write your own name. That's the reality for people with aphasia, a crippling disability that affects a third of the people who have a stroke every year. Strokes kill about one in twelve men and one in eight women, and are the third leading cause of death after heart disease and cancer. If you survive, a stroke can leave you with physical or mental disability.

Reducing your risk really does come down to some straightforward changes so it's worth finding out what you need to do. And some are even fun (such as drinking wine).

Here's an idea for you...

Eat a banana a day – it's the richest source of potassium, which helps reduce blood pressure, a major risk factor for strokes. Why not try a banana smoothie for breakfast? Blend a banana with some milk and bio-yogurt and add a teaspoon of honey to taste. Delicious.

Just like any organ in the body, the brain receives its blood supply via a network of vessels. Through these, the bloodstream feeds the brain with the oxygen and nutrients it needs for normal function. But when one or more vessels fail to supply enough blood to the brain, it may be damaged. This is what we know as a stroke, and it's why high cholesterol isn't just bad news for your heart. Clogged up arteries also affect the brain and increase your risk of stroke.

Now, back to that wine drinking. Moderate alcohol consumption helps to thin the blood and increase levels of healthy HDL cholesterol in the body, reducing your risk of stroke by about 20%. Keeping stress levels down is also thought to be important so why not wind down at the end of the day with a glass of wine? But note the word *moderate* – too much alcohol (more than two or three units a day) actually increases the risk.

Follow that glass of wine with a home-cooked, fish-based meal. Like alcohol, the oils found in fatty fish such as salmon, trout, tuna, mackerel and herring can increase HDL cholesterol levels. Eat fish five or more times each week and you'll have half the risk of suffering a stroke compared to people eating fish less than once a month.

Make sure you add a large serving of steamed mixed vegetables and maybe some brown rice to that fish to reduce your homocysteine levels. An increased amount of this naturally occurring substance in the body has been linked with a higher risk of heart disease. Now it's thought that it could also increase your chances of having a stroke. Certain nutrients, mainly vitamins B6, B12 and folic acid, have the ability to reduce homocysteine levels. So a good intake of these – by eating a diet high in fresh vegetables and wholegrains and by taking a daily B complex supplement – may help reduce the risk of stroke.

Eating too much salt can raise your blood pressure, which triples your risk of having a stroke whatever your age. For easy ways to cut back, see IDEA 16, Foods to lose.

Try another idea...

Whatever you do, don't cover your food with salt before you eat it. If you want to minimise your risk of stroke you should avoid adding salt during cooking or at the table, and also cut down on processed and fast foods. Salt increases the blood pressure which is thought to be the major risk factor for stroke. Products deceptively high in salt include canned soup, canned beans, cheese, processed meats, olives, mustard and soy sauce.

Finally, wash your meal down with a large glass of mineral water. At least two studies have found that magnesium intake from water appears to reduce the risk of stroke, so there is every possibility that drinking magnesium-rich mineral water may help to protect us in the long term.

'Minds, like bodies, will often fall into a pimpled, ill-conditioned state from mere excess of comfort.'
Charles Dickens

Defining idea...

How did it go?

Q   I read that Sharon Stone had a stroke because she was exercising too hard. Should I give up my circuit class, then?

A   *Definitely not! Regular exercise reduces high blood pressure, one of the major risk factors of stroke. It was widely but incorrectly reported in the press that Sharon Stone collapsed with a stroke while exercising at the gym. In fact, she admitted herself to hospital with a severe headache where they discovered bleeding between the brain and the skull due to a burst blood vessel. While she was young to suffer a stroke, it's thought to be on the increase in women who take oral contraceptive pills and smoke. One of the best things you can do to reduce your risk is to exercise regularly. So stick with the circuit class!*

Q   Is it possible to have a stroke and not realise you've had one?

A   *In theory. So-called 'silent strokes' occur when smaller blood vessels in the brain become blocked. Although they don't cause classic symptoms, they can increase the risk of them in the future. You can also have what is known as a mini-stroke, where you experience a few mild effects which improve in a short time (sometimes only minutes or hours). Your best bet is to reduce your risk of stroke with a healthy diet and lifestyle, then be aware of the main stroke symptoms and never ignore them. The most common symptoms are sudden numbness or weakness of the face, arm or leg, especially on one side of the body; sudden confusion, trouble speaking or understanding; sudden trouble seeing in one or both eyes; sudden trouble walking, dizziness, loss of balance or coordination or sudden, severe headache with no known cause. Seek medical help immediately if you have any of these symptoms – the sooner you receive treatment, the less long-term damage is done.*

43

Brain gym

A youthful body is nothing without a youthful mind, so it's time to give it a workout.

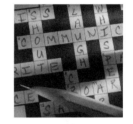

There's no point in working hard to fend off ageing and live a long and healthy life if you forget to look after your brain...

You're standing at the top of the stairs, wracking your brain for the reason you went up there in the first place. Or you meet a former work colleague on the street and can't for the life of you remember their name. Even if you don't get Alzheimer's (and two in every hundred people over the age of 65 will), if you don't exercise your brain as you age, like any muscle, it'll grow flabby.

The classic advice is to do a crossword a day. It's thought that keeping mentally active forces the brain to make new connections between cells. But did you know that one of the most effective ways to stay sharp is to exercise regularly? It all comes down to oxygen. Although the brain is only 2% of the body's weight, it consumes a quarter of your oxygen intake. When you use a particular part of the brain, the flow of oxygenated blood to that region (and therefore of oxygen) increases by 30%.

Looking for a new hobby? Take up tango dancing: scientists have specifically identified it as an activity which reduces the risk of developing Alzheimer's by an astonishing 75%. It seems this activity demands an unusual combination of multi-tasking, mixing mental and physical activity, thereby helping to maintain a robust hippocampus.

Defining idea...

'I always have trouble remembering three things: faces, names and – I can't remember what the third thing is.'
Fred A Allen, comedian

So anything that increases the flow of oxygen into the body – such as exercise – increases the brain's efficiency. You've probably noticed that a brisk walk around the block does wonders for speeding up your thought processes at work, or that the solution to a tricky problem can seem obvious after you've been for a run. Aim for around thirty minutes of moderate activity such as walking, swimming, cycling or jogging three times a week for best results.

A good diet will also help you keep on top of your game. Because the brain uses so much oxygen, it's a prime target for free radicals, the damaging by-product of the body's oxidation (oxygen-burning) process. Be sure to eat a high-antioxidant diet which includes a lot of fruit and vegetables, wholegrains and nuts. And watch how much you drink – excessive drinking can lead to loss of memory and reduced mental agility. You've probably noticed yourself that work and even simple daily tasks are much harder with a hangover. It's partly because alcohol attacks the body's store of glycogen, the brain's main energy source. But studies using brain scans have also shown that a hangover causes a depression in the cortex of the brain that coordinates your motor and auditory responses. So stick to a maximum of two or three drinks a day and have a couple of alcohol-free days every week.

There's truth in the old wives' tale that fish is brain food. See IDEA 11, Get hooked on fish, for ways to eat more.

Try another idea...

Now, back to those crosswords. Challenging your brain mentally is vital for living a youthful life for longer. There's no truth in the saying that you can't teach an old dog new tricks – an ageing brain is just as able to learn as a young one. Mental challenges, such as word puzzles, taking up a new hobby or learning a foreign language, keep neural connections strong, just as physical exercise keeps muscle fibres strong. Try simply shaking up one routine each day; take a new route home or use your non-dominant hand to brush your teeth, eat or apply cosmetics.

Got five minutes? Then you've time to boost your brain power with some simple exercises. Think up twenty uses for a toothpick or elastic band. Write a set of instructions for an everyday task, such as tying your shoelaces. Look inside your wardrobe for a few minutes, then shut the door. Make a descriptive list of everything inside. How much did you remember? You can try this with a painting or photograph. Practise using both hands at once. Bounce two balls, stir two cups of tea. Try throwing two wads of paper at a basket, one overhand, one underhand – simultaneously. It's a case of use it or lose it.

'There is a fountain of youth: it is your mind, your talents, the creativity you bring to your life and the lives of the people you love. When you learn to tap into this source, you will truly have defeated age.'
Sophia Loren

Defining idea...

Q I keep forgetting where I've left my keys or parked the car. Am I getting Alzheimer's?

A *Not necessarily. You can also become forgetful when you're stressed or depressed, or if you're deficient in vitamin B12. There's also a chance that you've actually always been this forgetful, except now that you're afraid it's a symptom of mental decline, you pay more attention to it. But do see your doctor if you start to feel disorientated, have problems performing difficult tasks or suffer unusual mood swings.*

Q I've got the option of retiring next year but I don't feel old. Should I give up work?

A *Definitely not, if you're still enjoying it. Some people think that forcing people to retire is the worst thing we can do for their mental health. Nowadays, more and more people are choosing not to retire at all – like Michael DeBakey, the pioneering heart surgeon who carried on operating into his nineties. If you still enjoy your work, and it's not causing you stress on a regular basis, you'll probably stay younger for longer by postponing that retirement bash for a few years.*

44

Bone up

Nothing says instant youth like a strong, supple spine – and it could add years to your life.

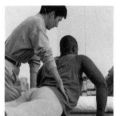

It's time for your skeleton to come out of the cupboard. It's hidden away so it's easy to forget about — until something goes wrong.

A fracture, or neck or back pain, can seriously restrict your plans to take up sand-yachting when you retire. A crumbling spine is also why some people shrink as they get older. Losing an inch or so in height can be expensive when you have to get all your trousers taken up!

Our bones do naturally become weaker with age, but they should remain strong enough to support us as long as we're alive. However, in some people the skeleton starts crumbling at a faster than normal rate, leading to osteoporosis. It affects one third of all women but don't think you're immune if you've never worn a skirt – one in twelve men are also at risk.

The bones in our skeleton are made of a thick outer shell and a strong inner mesh filled with collagen (protein), calcium salts and other minerals. The inside looks like

Here's an idea for you...

Is your bed giving you backache? Here's a simple way to tell. Lie on your back and slide your hand (palm down) into the small of your back. If there is a large gap, the mattress is too hard. If you have to squeeze your hand in, then it is too soft. If your hand slides in fairly easily, the mattress is just right.

honeycomb, with blood vessels and bone marrow in the spaces between bone. Osteoporosis occurs when the holes between the honeycomb become bigger, making it fragile and liable to break easily. Osteoporosis usually affects the whole skeleton but it most commonly causes fractures in the wrist, spine and hip.

But the good news is that bone is alive and constantly changing. Old, worn out bone is broken down and replaced by bone-building cells, called osteoblasts. This process of renewal is called bone turnover. And there's much you can do to increase your bone turnover and improve your bone strength – whatever your age.

Eating a bone-friendly diet is your first step. You probably already know that calcium is essential. You need around 700–1000 mg a day, which you could get from having, say, a half a pint of semi-skimmed milk, a low-fat yogurt, and a pot of low-fat cottage cheese in a day. Non-dairy sources of calcium include green leafy vegetables, baked beans, dried fruit and oily fish such as sardines, pilchards or anchovies where you eat the bones. You can also get it from tap water if you live in a hard water area – a bonus to make up for years of descaling your kettle!

Defining idea...

'I will never give in to old age until I become old. And I'm not old yet!'
Tina Turner

If you'd like to make sure you're getting enough calcium, consider taking a daily calcium supplement. Look for one that contains vitamin D, which helps the body absorb calcium. And on the subject of supplements, make sure you're not taking too much vitamin A. Recent research has suggested it may increase the risk of broken bones. Watch out if you take a multivitamin and a cod liver oil supplement which tend to be high in vitamin A. Try switching to a fish oil, rather than a fish *liver* oil, supplement instead (vitamin A is stored in the liver of fish). You shouldn't be getting more than 1500 mg of vitamin A a day.

And although it may seem like the last thing you should do if your bones are weak, do some exercise. Putting repetitive 'stress' on the bones stimulates new bone formation. Swimming or cycling won't help – it needs to be weight-bearing exercise, such as walking, jogging, aerobics or dancing.

Lifting weights is not just great for muscles – it also strengthens your bones. Find out the easiest way to do it at IDEA 24, *Pump some iron.*

Try another idea...

'I like long walks, especially when they are taken by people who annoy me.'
Fred A Allen, comedian

Defining idea...

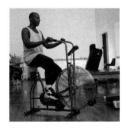 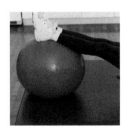 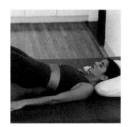

How did it go?

Q   My posture has definitely got worse as I've got older. How can I remember to stand up straight?

A   *It's worth paying a bit of attention to it because poor posture is instantly ageing – not only does slumping compress the spine, making you look shorter than your full height, it can also push the pelvis forwards, leaving us with a pot belly. It can also lead to neck and back pain, migraine headaches and even breathing and digestion problems. Simply thinking 'loose' and 'tall' in everything you do is a good start. All movements start from the brain, so just thinking about walking tall can send the right signals to your muscles. Imagine there's a balloon attached to your head, floating to the ceiling and taking your head with it. And try not to lean forward when you walk – look ahead, not down at the ground.*

Q   I've heard you can get a scan to check your bones. How do I know if I need one?

A   *A bone density or DXA scan is used to measure the density of bones and compare this to a normal range. See your doctor to discuss whether you should have one if you've broken a bone after a minor fall, had an early menopause (before the age of 45), an early hysterectomy (before the same age) or have had missing periods in the past for six months or more (excluding pregnancy) as a result of over-exercising or over-dieting. Long-term use of high dose corticosteroid tablets, for conditions such as arthritis and asthma, or a close family history of osteoporosis, particularly if your mother suffered a hip fracture, may also increase your risk.*

45

Keeping abreast

Going for a walk every day could be the best thing you do for the health of your breasts.

Exercise is something we all intend to do – tomorrow. A busy life has a habit of getting in the way of exercising. But if you want that life to continue as long as possible, you've got to make room for some exercise.

Whatever it takes – throwing away the TV, getting up half an hour earlier, giving up ironing clothes – your number one priority to yourself, if you want to be healthy for longer, is to exercise regularly.

Women tend to associate exercise with being skinny, so when you've hit 30 and realised that the key to a happy life is not fitting into a smaller-sized dress, it's easy to ditch the gym along with the fad diets. But the truth is that as you get older exercise gets even more vital. Done on a regular basis, it's one of the most effective ways of staving off breast cancer, the most common cancer in women.

Here's an idea for you... **Why not sign up for a charity fun-run? There are hundreds of women-only walking or running races held in aid of breast cancer research every year. It's a definite win–win situation – you'll reduce your chances of getting breast cancer by training for the race and you'll help to raise funds for research into the bargain.**

Let's have some good news – deaths from breast cancer have fallen by 20% over the past decade. But it still affects around one in nine women at some point and your chances of getting it increase with age. But just half an hour of brisk walking a day can reduce your risk by up to 30%. It used to be thought that only intense exercise such as jogging or aerobics decreased the risk, but now the latest research suggests that moderate activities such as walking, cycling or swimming also count. Even a couple of brisk walks a week will make a big difference.

But you'll only benefit from this effect if you're not overweight. It's thought that excess weight increases levels of hormones and growth factors (like oestrogen and insulin) that promote cancer development and that exercise can't counter these effects. But that's no reason to throw away your trainers if you know you need to lose some flab. Doing around thirty minutes of moderate exercise daily will help you lose weight and keep it off. Combine that with a diet high in plant foods – vegetables, fruits, wholegrains, pulses – and moderate amounts of oily fish, and low amounts of meat and saturated fat, and you could further reduce your risk by up to 33%.

Defining idea... *'The secret to staying young is to live honestly, eat slowly, and lie about your age.'* Lucille Ball

And a word of warning. The link between drinking and breast cancer makes sobering reading. One glass a day is fine and if you choose a dark red wine, you'll be getting an antioxidant boost into the bargain. But regularly drinking more than two units of alcohol a day can increase your risk of breast cancer by 40%. It's thought that alcohol interferes with the enzymes that break down oestrogen. If girls' nights out on the town are a thing of a past, it can be easy to assume your drinking is fine. But you also need to keep track of those generous glasses of wine you pour at home. One glass of most wines is around a unit, but that's a 125 ml wine glass. Try to stick to no more than two glasses a night, and have two alcohol-free nights a week. If this doesn't sound like much fun, then think of it another way. If you cut back on quantity you can afford to upgrade the quality – and savour every delicious drop.

Women who eat a lot of soy have a lower rate of breast cancer. For ideas on how to eat more soy, see IDEA 14, *The joy of soy*.

Try another idea...

Q I'm now inspired to check my breasts regularly. What's the best routine?

How did it go?

A *Doctors have moved on and now no longer recommend a specific routine for breast checking. Instead, they encourage you to simply get to know your breasts. Which may sound a bit odd – but they're not expecting you to look down and say, 'Hi, how do you do?'. It's about giving some attention to an area of your body you may take for granted. Which is why you should get your partner in on the act. Both of you should be aware of any changes, rather than just lumps. Any kind of thickening of the breast, change in shape or size, dimpling or puckering of the skin, or a change in the appearance of a nipple should be checked out with your doctor.*

199

Q My mum has just been diagnosed with breast cancer. Does that mean I'll get it?

A   *Not at all. Only 4% of breast cancer cases are thought to be genetically linked. The rest are caused by lifestyle factors – which is something you can do something about. But a very small number of women are at especially high risk because of faulty genes known as BRCA1 and BRCA2. If other family members have developed the disease, especially before the age of 50, see your doctor.*

Q Is it possible for men to get breast cancer?

A   *Yes, it is, although it's rare. Each year, there are around 200–300 cases of male breast cancer in the UK. This compares with about 40,500 cases of female breast cancer. The same rules apply about being aware of changes in the chest area and reporting them to your doctor.*

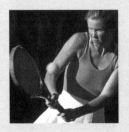 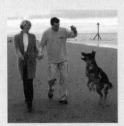 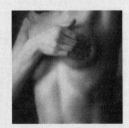

46

For men only

Real men do take care of their health – and even go to the doctor – if they want to live longer.

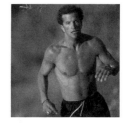

We all know that men and women were created equal — except, that is, when it comes to living longer.

Women outlive men by nearly six years and the gender gap is getting wider. Doctors think hormones may have a part to play. During their reproductive years, women are much less likely than men to suffer from heart disease, because their high levels of oestrogen lower LDL (bad) cholesterol and raise HDL (good) cholesterol. (After the menopause, when oestrogen levels drop, heart disease becomes the leading cause of death in women as well as men). It's thought that oestrogen can also help to protect women from stroke and colon cancer.

It's unlikely that men would queue up for artificial doses of oestrogen to help them live longer. But there are many lifestyle changes that you can make that will help you live as long as women. Giving up smoking is the first one – for all the media hype about teenage girls taking up smoking, the biggest group of smokers is still

If it's been a while since you saw your doctor, write down a list of all the concerns you'd raise in your ideal, fantasy consultation. Now, choose the most important of these concerns, make an appointment and talk it through thoroughly. You'll get the most out of your appointment if you focus on one problem rather than listing a raft of niggles. Try writing any questions you have before you get there, and make a note of the main symptoms, when they first appeared, and what, if any, medication you've used to treat it in the past.

men. Drinking is another concern. Despite all the news coverage about women becoming binge drinkers, heavy drinking – which increases the incidence of hypertension, stroke, liver disease, accidents and various cancers – is still most prevalent in men. (Have you ever walked into a local bar and found it full of solitary female drinkers? Probably not.)

Men also eat fewer vegetables than women. And when overweight, they tend to carry the weight on their stomachs, becoming the classic apple shape, unlike women, who carry it on their hips and thighs. Fat stored in the abdominal region is associated with an increased risk of heart disease.

But perhaps the biggest factor of all is that women take better preventative care of themselves than men. They spend more time finding out about health, and are more likely to notice symptoms and report them to their doctor. According to research, when men finally do get themselves to the doctor, they are more likely to play down their symptoms – and then ignore the advice given.

Defining idea...

'Old age is like everything else. To make a success of it, you've got to start young.'
Fred Astaire

It's time to abandon the macho mentality that real men don't go to the doctor. If it's the white coat that makes you feel uncomfortable, next time you walk past your surgery, walk in and pick up a leaflet about the services on offer. Most surgeries now offer a team of experts and range of services, so you may be able to get your problem sorted without even seeing a doctor. The practice nurse, for example, can test your blood pressure and cholesterol level or deal with other routine matters, often in a drop-in clinic. Some medical centres also have physiotherapists, counsellors and even specialist 'well man' clinics. Remember, it's your taxes that are funding these services so get out there and make the most of them!

You don't think twice about getting your car serviced, so why skimp on your body? Check out the checks you need at IDEA 52, *Check it out!*

Try another idea...

'If you compare all the major killers, such as heart disease and lung cancer, men easily come out best, from the undertaker's point of view.'
Dr Ian Banks, Chairman of the Men's Health Forum

Defining idea...

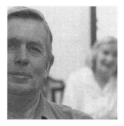
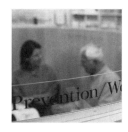
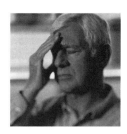

How did it go?

Q   I've been feeling a bit odd recently. Is it true that there's a male menopause?

A   *It's true that levels of the male hormone testosterone decline with age and that at 80, you'll have half the testosterone you had at 20. But it's a very slow, steady decline that starts around the age of 40 so it shouldn't produce any specific symptoms in the way that the female menopause does. However, some experts believe that levels can drop more rapidly than normal in some men, resulting in symptoms such as fatigue, a low mood, irritability, lack of energy and concentration. You may find you're not performing so well at work – or in the bedroom. Bear in mind that these symptoms can also be caused by lifestyle factors such as being overweight and unfit, drinking too much and having a poor diet. But if you're otherwise pretty healthy, and your symptoms come on suddenly, your best bet is to discuss it with your doctor who may decide you need hormone tests.*

Q   My father had prostate cancer so I make sure I get the right checks. But what else can I do to make sure I don't get it too?

A   *Eat more tomatoes for a start – an antioxidant found in tomatoes, called lycopene, seems to fight off cancer cells in the prostate. Before you rush off and munch your way through a bag of tomatoes, bear in mind that the body cannot absorb lycopene except in the presence of fat. So simply drinking a glass of tomato juice won't help but eating tomato pastes and sauces which contain a little oil will – and that includes ketchup! Alternatively, warm up some tinned plum tomatoes for breakfast and have them on buttered toast, drizzle fresh tomatoes with olive oil in a salad, or mix fresh tomatoes with sun-dried tomatoes in oil. An added bonus could be healthier arteries – men and women with high levels of lycopene in the bloodstream also have healthy arteries.*

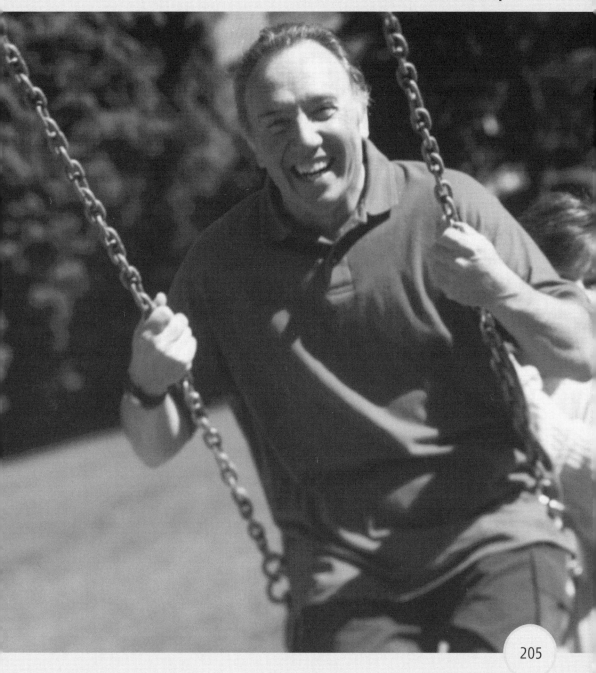

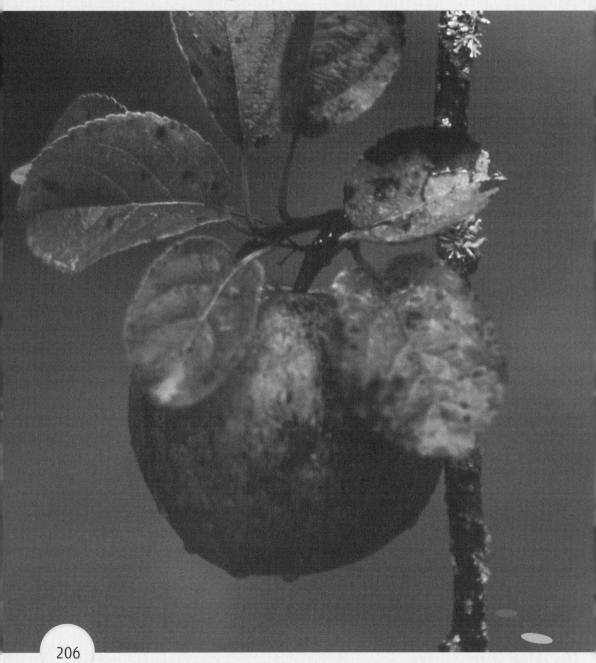

47

The last taboo?

We're so coy about our bodily functions that bowel cancer cuts short the lives of thousands of people every year.

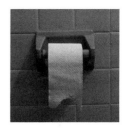

We shouldn't be. If it's caught early, colon cancer can be cured.

There's nothing some people enjoy more than a bit of toilet humour, but getting anyone to seriously discuss their bowel habits is a completely different matter. In these days of fly-on-the-wall documentaries and reality television shows, it's easy to think there are no more taboos. But one of the biggest ones of all is what goes on behind the bathroom door.

Just a mention of the word bottom or toilet can often produce a snigger from somewhere. But what's revealing is that while cancer of the colon is the third most common cancer in men, and the second most common cancer in women, no one holds fashion shows, nor are there sales of pretty coloured ribbons, in aid of colon cancer research. It's just not glamorous.

Here's an idea for you...

They say you should never look back, but here's when you should. Next time you go to the loo, take a good look before you flush. A black, tarry substance means blood is leaking into your system – which could be a sign of a stomach ulcer or bowel cancer. You should also look out for bright red flecks. Don't panic if you do spot some; there are other causes of bleeding than cancer. But always see your doctor.

So here's some basic information. Bowel cancer is caused by damage to the genes involved in the growth and survival of cells lining the bowel. Most bowel cancers start as a small growth in the lining of the bowel called a polyp. Polyps are normally harmless but can turn cancerous.

One of the biggest risk factors is being a sufferer of a chronic bowel condition, such as ulcerative colitis or Crohn's disease, a condition of inflammation and ulceration in the small intestine. Around one in twenty cases develop in someone with a strong family history of bowel cancer.

If you don't have either of these conditions, but you do have a serious steak and burger habit, you're also at risk. A diet that is high in red and processed meat is thought to be one of the biggest risk factors. Eating a diet rich in fibre, fruit and vegetables is the best start to reducing the risk, but if you've been used to a 'meat and two veg' kind of eating, changing the habits of a lifetime won't be easy.

You do have lot of options, however, and they are worth exploring. Why not swap a few of your usual lamb, beef or pork dishes for poultry or fish, or even bean or lentil dishes? Eating the skin of baked potatoes isn't a hardship, and that's high in fibre, as is wholemeal bread – use that instead of white. Make small changes like those, and get used to them gradually, then soon you won't miss your red meat as much as you thought you would.

Your bowels will thank you for eating more porridge. See IDEA 15, *Porridge power*.

Try another idea...

And if you have a family history of bowel cancer, see your doctor about screening. Before you say, 'I don't want any doctor sticking his hand up my bottom,' that won't happen. These days diagnosis involves gently pushing a long thin tube containing a tiny video camera into the rectum and colon to see what's going on. While this isn't most people's idea of fun, it doesn't hurt.

Remember, if caught early, colon cancer is 90% curable. So don't be shy. If you notice any sudden changes in your bowel habit, such as looser or more frequent stools, bleeding that's not due to piles or unexplained anaemia, see your doctor. It's simple. The older you get, the more attention you need to pay to your behind!

'You do live longer with bran, but you spend the last fifteen years on the toilet.'
Alan King, comedian

Defining idea...

How did it go?

Q **Sometimes I don't have a bowel movement for days. Is this normal?**

A *Most of us assume that once a day is 'normal', although our digestive system, like that of all primates, is designed to eliminate solid waste a few times a day. If you're not moving your bowels for days, try drinking more water. Being dehydrated is one of the commonest causes of constipation. Aim for eight glasses a day. Base the bulk of your diet on fresh fruit and vegetables by aiming for your five portions a day, and eat wholegrain bread and pasta, and brown rice. There's also a psychological aspect to constipation: if you don't feel comfortable with the toilet facilities available, such as at work or when you're out enjoying yourself, you may be unconsciously 'holding on'. Try to relax and go to the toilet as soon as you feel a need. Remember, everyone does it!*

Q **I've never felt right in the toilet department. Does this mean I'm destined to have bowel cancer?**

A *Not necessarily. You could be suffering from irritable bowel syndrome, a digestive disorder thought to affect as many as one in ten people. With IBS, the bowel is abnormally sensitive, so the passage of food can cause pain and discomfort. Symptoms include constipation, diarrhoea, wind, bloating, abdominal pain and nausea. If this sounds familiar, see your doctor. As yet there is no cure for IBS, but treatments include following a special diet, relaxation therapies such as hypnotherapy to reduce stress, medication to control diarrhoea, laxatives for constipation and antispasmodic drugs for abdominal pain. Some people have found complementary therapies useful.*

48

Saving your senses

The future's bright, so here's what you need to do today to make sure you can see – and hear – it for longer!

Does reading the newspaper these days hurt your arms — because you have to hold it at arms' length to read it? Do you only like reading where there's a bright light available?

This is regarded as part of the eyes' normal ageing process and is known as presbyopia. Normal, healthy, young eyes have a wide range of focus from the far distance to a few centimetres. In a young eye, the lens is very flexible. As we get older, the lens of the eye thickens and slowly loses its flexibility leading to a gradual decline in our ability to focus on objects that are close up. It's why many of us need reading glasses from the age of 40 onwards.

But there's also a theory that the loss of focusing ability in later life is mainly due to acquired habits of strain which can be both prevented and reversed. According to American ophthalmologist Dr William Bates, some simple exercises can help. The theory is that vision problems aren't static and can be improved by keeping the eye muscles relaxed and moving freely. Exercises include spending time with your palms over your eyes every day, and choosing a different colour on each day of the

If you're having trouble hearing, get your ears syringed! Hearing is often dulled by ears full of wax. You can get drops over the counter from a pharmacy to soften the wax. Use it for a week then book an appointment with the nurse at your doctor's surgery to have your ears syringed. You may well be amazed at just how much better you can hear afterwards.

week and consciously looking out for that colour all day. For more information on the Bates method, see www.seeing.org.

But there are more serious eye conditions to avoid as you age. Age-related macular degeneration (or AMD for short) and cataracts are the leading causes of blindness in the developed world. AMD affects 20% of people over the age of 65 and cataracts almost 50% of those over 75. But both could be avoided by simply eating more vegetables.

Many people grew up with their mothers saying 'Eat up your carrots, they'll help you see in the dark'. It's just one of the many old wives' tales that have finally been proved true by scientific research. It makes you wonder where those old wives got such accurate insight before laboratories, white coats and doctors were even invented! But that's another story. We now know that the beta-carotene contained in carrots can convert into vitamin A, which has a critical role to play in night vision. We also know that your mother should have added, 'and while you're at it, finish off your dark green vegetables, pumpkin and red peppers'!

Defining idea...

'Keep your eyes on the stars, and your feet on the ground.'
Theodore Roosevelt

These vegetables are all high in a micronutrient called lutein, which helps to stave off the free radical damage thought to cause AMD. Boosting your intake of disease-fighting carotenoids in dark green and orange-yellow vegetables such as carrots, spinach, broccoli and squash will also help. Foods rich in carotenoids (especially spinach, kale and broccoli) will also help you fend off cataracts, as will vitamins C (from fruits and veg) and E (found in vegetable oils, nuts and seeds, egg yolks and green leafy vegetables). If you're a fan of the 'belt-and-braces' approach, up your vegetable intake, and take a daily multivitamin supplement. It could reduce your long-term cataract risk by 60%, according to one study.

Drinking a little wine may also help reduce your risk of AMD. See IDEA 13, *The good news about booze.*

Try another idea...

Hearing is also a vital sense for keeping us in touch with the world around us. Many people find their hearing becoming less acute once they are past the age of 50, and a majority of those over 70 have some degree of hearing loss. This happens as the cochlea in the inner ear become less effective at picking up sound, especially high-pitched ones. Most experts now agree that people could avoid long-term hearing loss by simply avoiding loud noises. If you refuse to give up those heavy metal concerts, at least wear earplugs. And never be tempted to leave off your protective ear muffs if you work in a noisy environment.

Your hearing will not normally be tested at a routine check-up but if you suspect it has deteriorated, your doctor may do some preliminary tests or refer you for specialist investigation.

'Of all the senses, sight must be the most delightful.'
Helen Keller, who was both blind and deaf

Defining idea...

How did it go?

Q   I can't really follow a conversation in a noisy environment any more but I really don't want to wear a hearing aid. What else can I do?

A   *Unfortunately there is no cure for the age-related decline in hearing but hearing aids can make a world of difference. Are memories of an ancient uncle whose hearing aid used to whistle away putting you off? Technology has moved on massively and today's devices are silent, and so tiny they're undetectable. Of course, avoiding places with lots of background noise such as bars and restaurants can help. But if you're also finding it difficult to follow a conversation in any social environment, see your doctor for a referral to a hearing specialist. Cutting yourself off from socialising is one of the fastest ways to speed up the ageing process.*

Q   I don't want to wear reading glasses. Don't they make your eyes lazy?

A   *I'm afraid this is a bit of a myth. While to a certain extent you do 'get used' to wearing glasses, it's a case of getting used to not straining in order to see and being able to read without effort. But if you hate the idea of having reading glasses, you're in luck – you can now get bifocal contact lenses, individually prescribed for each person's special combination of distance and near vision. It means that reading small print – as well as shifting focus between the road and a car's speedometer – becomes a lot easier.*

49

The accident factor

Accidents can happen anywhere, while you're doing anything from driving to DIY.

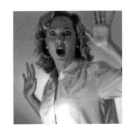

Most are entirely preventable; here's how to minimise the risk.

You may be wondering what accidents have to do with living longer, apart from the fact that a serious accident can cause premature death. On average, in industrialised countries – and also in many developing countries – one hospital bed in ten is occupied by someone who has been involved in an accident.

And accidents that don't kill you can age you; injuries can make you less mobile and active, and they can also cause you stress – your immune system's greatest enemy. But most accidents can be easily prevented, with a little care and forethought.

Take DIY. Your home is your sanctuary but it can also be a dangerous place to be if you're not careful. DIY is a particular danger point. Why is it that we blithely attempt jobs involving old, wobbly ladders and power tools without wearing the right clothes or taking any safety preparations – such as getting someone to hold the ladder? If you're planning to do some work around the house, make sure you invest in the right safety gear such as thick gloves, goggles and a good ladder (get rid of that old rickety one, or you may still be tempted to use it). And place it on a firm surface.

Don't rely on your sense of smell alone to detect dangerous odours such as smoke around the home. Fit smoke and carbon monoxide alarms this week if you haven't already done so. If you have, check the batteries and change any that need replacing. Don't 'borrow' the batteries from the alarm for something else and forget to replace them!

And it's not a good idea to hire power tools that you know little about; things are not always as easy to use as they may appear to be on television makeover programmes. Don't do DIY if you're tired or short on time, and therefore likely to rush and cut corners. It isn't worth it.

Ancient ladders aside, falls account for many accidents in the home, and are one of the biggest causes of death among those aged 65–74. You're more likely to suffer a fall if you're unfit; weak muscles can't recover quickly if you stumble or trip. However, you can minimise your risk by storing things you use frequently at easy-to-reach height, keeping the floor clear of clutter and making sure you have good lighting in your home, particularly in stair areas.

Defining idea... **'Accidents will occur in the best-regulated families.'**
Charles Dickens

Worldwide, car accidents kill an estimated one million people a year and, of course, not all are fatal. Road accidents are a major cause of severe injuries. Driving while tired is estimated to play a significant part in many accidents on motorways and fast roads. Research has also shown that sleep-related accidents are more likely to result in death or serious injuries than other types of road accident.

Accidents due to fatigue are most likely to occur between 4 a.m. and 6 a.m. – but the natural 'siesta' time of 2–4 p.m. is also a high-risk period. The length of time behind the wheel is not important – most accidents involving tired drivers occur during the first hour. So don't even attempt that trip to the local shops if you're feeling sleepy.

Strength training regularly can reduce your risk of falls. Find out the easiest ways to do it at IDEA 24, *Pump some iron.*

Try another idea...

Wearing a seat belt and having an airbag fitted to your car can greatly improve your chances of surviving an accident, as can slowing down – simply driving within five miles of the speed limit can add three years to your life.

Bizarrely, one of the other most risky places to spend time is in a hospital, where the MRSA bug can be picked up. MRSA is resistant to some antibiotics including penicillin; although it's harmless to most of us, it can override the immune system of anyone weakened by illness or surgery. You can reduce your risk of infection simply by washing your hands regularly while in hospital, and asking any staff who examine you to wash their hands first. And of course, cut down your risk of ending up there in the first place by avoiding accidents...

'There is no such thing as an accident; it is fate misnamed.'
Napoleon Bonaparte

Defining idea...

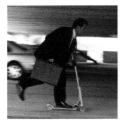 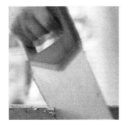

How did
it go?

Q   **I love skiing but can be prone to falling over. Should I give it up if I want to live longer?**

A   *Skiing's not as risky a sport as you might think. Statistics show that for every thousand people skiing per day, only between two and four will sustain an injury that requires medical attention. And there are simple ways to reduce your risk of injury, such as not skiing when you're tired and not attempting runs that are beyond your ability. Why not sign up for some more lessons on your next trip and see if you can fall over less? And in case you were wondering what the riskiest sports are, in terms of number of injuries, they're rugby and football – playing, not watching!*

Q   **I'm not really into DIY but I'm a keen gardener. But that's a nice safe hobby, isn't it?**

A   *Afraid not. Gardens are pretty risky places to be. Astonishingly, many people are injured actively gardening every year – but when you remember that electrical equipment is often involved, perhaps it's not so surprising. The most dangerous combination is a man with a mower. Other dangers include flowerpots (people trip or fall on them), secateurs and pruners, spades and electric hedgetrimmers. Always put on gloves, shoes and trousers when mowing the lawn rather than shorts and sandals, don't use a strimmer in sandals and only use electric mowers and other power tools that have an RCD – residual current device – which will cut off the power quickly in the event of an accident. Do use power breakers; it is very easy to strim or mow or even hedgetrim through a power cable, even if it is bright orange.*

50

Breath of life

Here's something you can do to stave off ageing right now. Take a deeper breath.

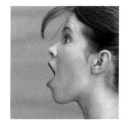

Some of the effects of ageing are unavoidable; they are there every time we look in the mirror. Others are easy to overlook.

On average we breathe 20,000 times a day. It's thought that as we get older, most of us experience a 20% reduction in blood oxygen levels caused by poor breathing habits. And as every cell in the body depends on oxygen for life, that has a big effect on our health and the rate at which we age.

You probably didn't even realise you had a breathing 'habit'. It's something we all do without thinking about most of the time. But a combination of poor posture, and weak or stiff muscles surrounding the lungs, can restrict the amount of oxygen we take in.

The result is a breathing pattern of short, shallow breaths known as hyperventilation. You may be hyperventilating if your chest, rather than your abdomen, moves with each breath, if you breathe faster than normal (more than

Here's an idea for you...

Want to know how deeply you breathe? Put your hands on your abdomen, just below the base of your rib cage, as you take your next breath in. If you're breathing deeply, your hands will move as your stomach expands. (We're all born breathing like this – watch a baby sleeping and you'll see its stomach rise and fall – but our breath becomes shallower as we age.) When the lungs are filled to capacity, they push down the diaphragm which causes the stomach to slightly expand. If your hands don't move, then take deeper, slower breaths until they do. Do this exercise on a regular basis until it becomes second nature.

fourteen breaths a minute) or you have a tendency to take big breaths before you speak, hold your breath mid-conversation or you do a lot of unconscious sighing or yawning throughout the day!

If it's a habit you've had for a long time, you may not even notice the effects. But it's thought that the overuse of the chest and neck muscles from overbreathing in this way can lead to muscle tension and pain. Hyperventilating can also lead to low levels of carbon dioxide in the blood which has been linked with irregular heartbeat, and not getting enough oxygen to the brain can make you feel tired, forgetful and irritable. Hyperventilaters also tend to have high blood pressure and there is even a theory, although not one held by the entire medical profession, that hyperventilation triggers asthma – by breathing too often, you breathe out too much carbon dioxide which causes the airways in the lungs to go into spasm, triggering the symptoms of asthma.

Hyperventilation does have a useful purpose – it's part of the fight or flight response designed to help us escape from danger. But constant hyperventilating means you're constantly sending the body signals that it's under stress. Not only is this disastrous for the immune system, it can also trigger panic attacks in some of us.

Many yoga classes concentrate on improving the breathing. For more good reasons to dust off your exercise gear, see IDEA 25, *Flexing your options*.

Try another idea...

But it is possible to retrain your breathing patterns; it will take time to change the habit of a lifetime, so don't expect instant results. Start by consciously trying to slow your breathing down to a rate of ten or twelve breaths per minute. The effort of breathing should come from your diaphragm not your chest – the chest should hardly move. And watch your posture – it's hard to breathe deeply if you're slumped. Standing straight, with your shoulders back, automatically opens up the chest area. Many people find that learning the Alexander Technique to improve posture also has a big effect on their breathing, which is why it's so popular with performers. You could also take singing lessons – learning to breathe from the diaphragm is an integral part. Who knows, as well as feeling calmer and more energised, you may even discover a new talent!

'He lives most life whoever breathes most air.'
Elizabeth Barrett Browning

Defining idea...

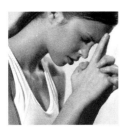
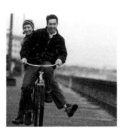

221

How did it go?

Q   My breathing is very shallow. How can I learn to breathe more deeply?

A   *Here's an easy exercise to help – try to do it twice a day. Sit up straight. Exhale, then inhale while trying to relax the belly muscles. Then imagine your belly filling with air. After filling the belly, keep inhaling. Think about the middle of your chest filling with air. Feel your chest and rib cage expand. Hold the breath in for a moment, then begin to exhale as slowly as possible. As the air is slowly let out, relax your chest and rib cage. Begin to pull your belly in to force out the remaining breath. Try to stay relaxed throughout and repeat for around five minutes.*

Q   I often feel short of breath. Does this mean I'm really unfit?

A   *Yes, if you become out of breath after even mild exertion such as climbing stairs, you need to prioritise time for exercise in your life in order to get your heart, lungs and muscles in better shape. But if you feel out of breath all the time, you could be an undiagnosed asthma sufferer. Other symptoms include wheezing and coughing, particularly at night. If this sounds familiar, make an appointment to see your doctor this week. If you feel breathless in stressful situations and also feel light-headed, you may be hyperventilating and suffering from panic attacks. Try to make a conscious effort to take long, slow deep breaths when you start to feel like this.*

51

Looking younger

We're all creatures of vanity at heart. When you look young, you feel young. Here's how to keep the visible signs of ageing at bay.

Creams, lotions, potions, injections, operations — there are trillions of ways to spend money on looking younger. The question is, do any of them work? Undoubtedly, some do.

In fact, if you're not phobic about needles and you've got a bit of spare cash to spend on yourself, there are lots of so-called 'lunch-hour' treatments now available that can make you look fresher and brighter in nearly an instant. The ever popular injections of Botox or botulinum toxin freeze facial muscles to smooth out furrows and prevent existing wrinkles deepening. You can also get your lines and wrinkles plumped out with artificial 'fillers' such as NewFill or Perlane, synthetic forms of hyaluronic acid, a natural substance that contributes to skin plumpness. Some people combine the two – injecting a filler into the wrinkle along with Botox – so the wrinkle is plumped out but also frozen at the same time to prevent it becoming any deeper. You can also have fillers injected into thinning lips to plump them out.

Here's an idea for you...

Start wearing sunscreen on your face every day. Most (80%) of the lines and wrinkles you see in the mirror are caused by the sun but it's never too late to prevent more damage. We now know it's the sun's UVA, or non-burning, rays that age the skin, which means you're affected even in winter. Many daily moisturisers now include sun protective ingredients – just make sure you opt for one that's 'broad spectrum', to block out both UVA and UVB rays. In summer months, wear a sunscreen specially formulated for the face instead.

One of the newest treatments is called fat transfer – where fat is removed from the thighs or bottom with liposuction and injected into the face to fill out lines and wrinkles. It's done under local anaesthetic; you can even freeze extra fat and come back for regular top-ups. A less drastic way to freshen up your face is microdermasion, where tiny 'sandblasting' crystals are used to scrub away surface imperfections and create all-over smoothness. It's great for skin that's been coarsened by too much sun exposure over the years. The next step up is laser skin resurfacing, which uses highly focused laser beams to vaporise the skin's upper layers and stimulate the formation of new collagen. Skin can be red and sore for up to a month afterwards so if you don't fancy a month in a mask, opt for a softer pulsed light treatment (such as Nlite) instead. It also encourages new collagen production, making wrinkles less prominent, but usually only causes soreness for a couple of hours afterwards.

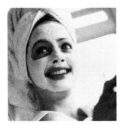

The main drawback with these treatments is the upkeep. Most need to be redone every three to six months, so if you like the effect, be prepared for an ongoing financial commitment to keep it up. A longer-lasting solution is to go under the knife, and there are lots of mini ops now available rather than the full facelift. You could just get your baggy eyes seen to (blepharoplasty), a procedure that's popular with men, or go for a lower face lift to get rid of a jowly jawline.

Eating a diet high in oily fish can stave off wrinkles according to some experts. Find out more at IDEA 11, *Get hooked on fish*.

Try another idea...

The key to success with all of these treatments is finding an experienced practitioner so always do your research before opting for any treatment. Botox should only be carried out by a properly qualified, medical, doctor, and fillers by specially trained nurses or doctors. Microdermasion and pulsed light treatments can be carried out by non-medically qualified staff so if possible, try to get a word-of-mouth recommendation. Stronger laser treatments should be carried out by a doctor.

We've all seen the pictures of Hollywood celebs who are refusing to get old and have had one treatment too many. But there's a difference between trying to look adolescent forever and wanting the face in the mirror to reflect how strong, youthful and energetic you feel inside. In the end, a zest for life, commitment to a healthy lifestyle and an openness to new ideas are your most vital weapons against ageing.

'Thirty-five is a very attractive age. London society is full of women of the highest birth who have, of their own free choice, remained thirty-five for years.'
Oscar Wilde

Defining idea...

How did
it go?

Q **My mother always said that over a certain age a woman must choose to keep her face or her figure. Any truth in this?**

A   It's a bit of an old wives' tale with a grain of truth in it. Losing fat from the face is a natural part of ageing, but if you lose a lot of weight suddenly, it will accelerate the process. Over the age of thirty, the skin can't adapt to sudden changes as it hasn't enough elasticity, so it starts to sag. But being overweight ages the body, so it's still best to shift the flab. Just aim for a steady loss of not more than a kilo (a couple of pounds) a week, and try to keep it level once you've reached your goal. Be sure to opt for a healthy, balanced diet – nothing shows up more on your face than poor nutrition.

Q **I'm a man so it's not so much my wrinkles I'm worried about as my thinning hair. What can I do about that?**

A   Whatever you do, avoid the comb-over. It fools no one. There are two topical treatments available that you apply to the scalp that seem to have some effect – minoxidil (sold as Regaine) and finasteride (sold as Propecia). Some men have found these products stopped hair loss, and even encouraged regrowth in those who are just beginning to lose hair. However, neither treatment is cheap and both require permanent usage for lasting results. Oh, and some men on Propecia experience a reduced desire for sex and difficulty in achieving an erection. If this sounds like hard work (pardon the pun), head for your barber instead and ask for a 'No. 1' all over. You'll instantly look ten years younger – not to mention trendy.

52

Check it out!

Ever fantasised about making an appointment with your doctor and saying, 'Check everything out, please'?

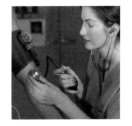

Getting a health all-clear is a great way to motivate you to maintain a healthier lifestyle in the future.

Regular health checks are essential if you want to live a long and healthy life because you've got a much better chance of curing many serious diseases – including cancer – if you catch them early. Unfortunately, doctors have neither the time nor the resources to run random tests for every patient, which leaves you with two options. You could opt for one of the many screening packages on offer from private health companies (which can be costly). Alternatively, there are many self-checks you can easily do at home which can help you assess whether you do really need to see your doctor for further investigation.

The first check is to find out if you're overweight or obese. Obesity is linked with a host of diseases such as cancer, diabetes and heart disease. To check if you're in the healthy weight range, calculate your body mass index (you'll probably need a calculator). First, measure your height in metres. Multiply this figure by itself (e.g. 1.5 m × 1.5 m). This gives your height squared. Now measure your weight in

Here's an idea for you...

If you don't know what your cholesterol level is, make an appointment with your doctor to get tested this week. Alternatively buy a cholesterol self-test from pharmacies which involves taking a small sample of blood from your finger tip and placing it on a test strip. Results are then compared to a colour chart in three minutes.

kilograms. Divide your weight by your height squared. This gives you your body mass index. A healthy figure is 20–25. A BMI of 25–30 is overweight; 30–40 is obese BMI, and above 40 is very obese. (If you don't want to do the maths, there's a BMI calculator on www.cyberdiet.com.)

If you are overweight, it's worth considering a diabetes test. The average person lives with diabetes for sixteen years before diagnosis – by which time the disease may have caused heart and kidney damage. You're more at risk if you have a family member with the disease, you're over fifty or overweight. You can buy a self-test for diabetes cheaply at most pharmacies, but be sure to follow it up with a medical appointment if it's positive.

Next, listen to your heartbeat. Heart disease is a massive killer, but you don't need to book in for an ECG (electrocardiogram) to check out your heart – simply observe what it's like after physical exertion such as climbing stairs. See your doctor if your heartbeat is irregular, or takes a long time to come back to normal.

If you've no idea what your blood pressure is, now's the time to find out. Hypertension, or high blood pressure, is the biggest cause of stroke or heart disease so it could be worth buying a digital blood pressure meter from pharmacies.

Now, some stuff for women only. Women over fifty are routinely invited for a mammogram every three years. But more than 90% of breast cancers are found by women themselves. The key is to be aware of what's normal for your breasts – don't get obsessive about checking them, but feel for any lumps once a month or so when you're in the bath or shower. And make sure you report anything unusual, such as nipple discharge or puckering of the skin of the breast, to your doctor.

When you're checking out your body, don't forget your teeth. Gum disease if left untreated can lead to heart disease. Find out how at IDEA 40, *Gum shield*.

Try another idea...

Also for women: don't skip your smear test. A smear test checks for cell changes on the cervix which could, if left untreated, lead to cervical cancer. Women aged between 20 and 64 should have a smear test every three to five years, although you may be tested more regularly if you have shown any signs of abnormal cells in the past. Men, meanwhile, should see their GP for a prostate test if they suddenly start peeing more frequently.

Checking your health doesn't have to be just another chore – it can even be fun if you rope in a partner. How about an all-over massage, with some mole checking thrown in? Look out for moles which have changed shape or colour, seem bigger, bleed or are itchy. Some men are also more than happy to take over checking their partner's breasts and also prefer their partners to check their testicles for unusual lumps that may be testicular cancer. Any excuse, eh, boys?

'Be careful about reading health books. You may die of a misprint.'
Mark Twain

Defining idea...

How did it go?

Q **I've been putting on weight lately and I swear I'm not eating any more than I used to. What test should I have?**

A *A thyroid function test could help. An underactive thyroid gland can be the root of gradual weight gain, especially in women over fifty, and if left untreated can lead to heart problems. Other symptoms include tiredness, feeling cold and losing the hair. A blood test from your doctor can show if your thyroid is functioning properly. Once it's ruled out, your doctor can decide if you need further tests.*

Q **Whatever disease I read about, I'm convinced I've got. My doctor is sick of the sight of me. What can I do?**

A *In years gone by, you'd simply be labelled a hypochondriac. But these days, we've got a new name for what you're suffering – health anxiety. It's thought to be on the increase thanks to an overload of information about health now available on the internet, on TV, in newspapers, magazines and books. The trouble is that many diseases – take diabetes for example – have symptoms which can also be caused by simply leading a stressful life. So it's easy to jump to wrong conclusions, but if you're doing this more and more often and feel like it's affecting your life, then see your doctor (again!). Explain what's happening; your doctor may decide to refer you to a cognitive behavioural therapist to help you get your fears into perspective.*

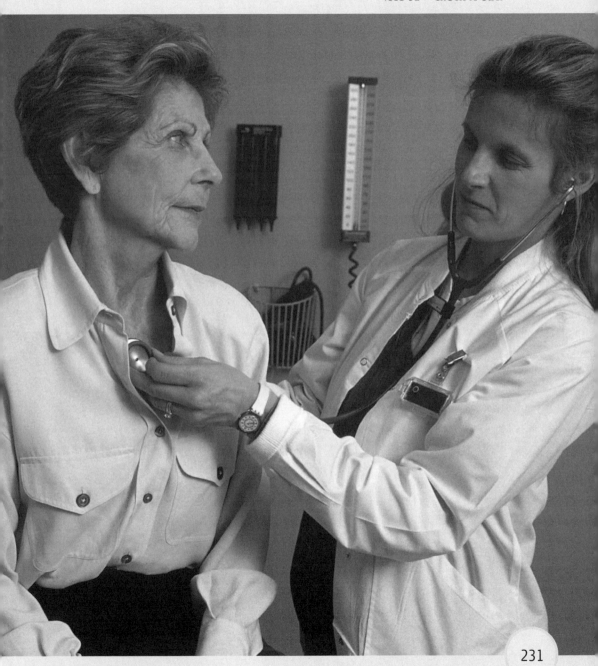

The end...

Or is it a new beginning?

We hope that the ideas in this book will have inspired you to try some new things to stay youthful. You should now be well on your way to living a longer, healthier life, packed with endless possibilities.

You're glowing and energetic and you don't care who knows it.

So why not let us know all about it? Tell us how you got on. What did it for you – what helped you to fight off the ageing process? Maybe you've got some tips of your own you want to share (see the next page if so). And if you liked this book you may find we have even more brilliant ideas that could change other areas of your life for the better.

You'll find the Infinite Ideas crew waiting for you online at www.infideas.com.

Or if you prefer to write, then send your letters to:
Live longer
The Infinite Ideas Company Ltd
36 St Giles, Oxford OX1 3LD, United Kingdom

We want to know what you think, because we're all working on making our lives better too. Give us your feedback and you could win a copy of another 52 Brilliant Ideas book of your choice. Or maybe get a crack at writing your own.

Good luck. Be brilliant.

Offer one

CASH IN YOUR IDEAS

We hope you enjoy this book. We hope it inspires, amuses, educates and entertains you. But we don't assume that you're a novice, or that this is the first book that you've bought on the subject. You've got ideas of your own. Maybe our author has missed an idea that you use successfully. If so, why not send it to info@infideas.com, and if we like it we'll post it on our bulletin board. Better still, if your idea makes it into print we'll send you £50 and you'll be fully credited so that everyone knows you've had another Brilliant Idea.

Offer two

HOW COULD YOU REFUSE?

Amazing discounts on bulk quantities of Infinite Ideas books are available to corporations, professional associations and other organizations.

For details call us on:
+44 (0)1865 514888
fax: +44 (0)1865 514777
or e-mail: info@infideas.com

Where it's at...

Even more brilliant ideas...

Lose weight and stay slim

Eve Cameron

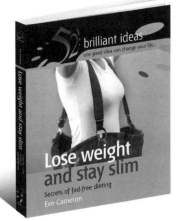

"Every week the media report on the latest fad diet that's sweeping Hollywood. Whether it's Atkins, food-combining or cabbage soup, there's always some new trend that promises to keep you slim. And yet at the same time we hear of an epidemic of obesity sweeping many parts of the world. It's pretty obvious that fad diets aren't working."

"That's why I've written this book. There are countless tricks and techniques I've learnt over the years to help you become and stay slim. Losing weight successfully and permanently requires both a lifestyle and mindset change, and that's what Lose weight and stay slim *offers you. Enjoy the new you!"* – **Eve Cameron**

Available from all good bookshops and online at www.amazon.co.uk

Whole health

Kate Cook

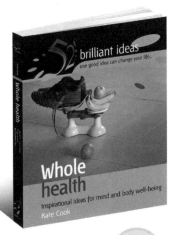

"The media seem to be obsessed with the deterioration of our physical and mental health. All you hear about is obesity, disease, binge drinking and drug addiction. And what's the usual answer?"

"Some complex detoxification programme, diets that mean you can only eat raw pulses and exercise regimes that will train you to be a marathon runner. Oh yes, and counselling so that your parents can ultimately take the blame for your problems."

"Here's a different approach that I've used myself and with friends and clients. It does involve exercise and diet but above all else – common sense! The net result will be a happier, healthier you."

Kate Cook

Control your blood pressure

Dr Rob Hicks

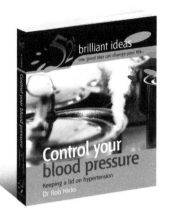

"High blood pressure affects nearly one in three women and two in five men and is a major contributor to strokes and heart disease."

The worst thing about it is that it rarely causes any symptoms. You may not know you're suffering from it until something bad happens, and by then it can be too late."

"But there's good news. By changing your lifestyle just a little you can become much healthier. And don't worry, I'm not advocating that you spend four hours a day in the gym, never touch alcohol again and eat only fresh vegetables! Just build into your daily life the practical advice in Control your blood pressure *and you can greatly reduce the risk of future problems. Staying healthy doesn't need to be a pain. You can get on top of your blood pressure and feel great in the process. Here's how!"* – **Dr Rob Hicks**

Available from all good bookshops and online at www.amazon.co.uk

Win at the gym

Steve Shipside

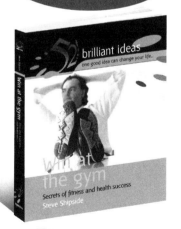

"I was so out of shape and overweight that my doctor told me I was well on my way to chronic back pain. I would have answered back but I was fully engaged in sucking my belly in at the time. I'm no superman and was never a natural gym bunny yet now I'm an Ironman triathlete and ultrarunner. That's despite having Better Things To Do (watching telly, washing up, anything really). On the way I've learnt that there is no marathon as grim and as glum as getting nowhere in the gym. If you've ever caught a glimpse of yourself in the gym mirrors and thought, 'what's the point?', then these are the ideas you need to go the distance, and get the results you want.

That's my story. This is yours. It starts here..." **Steve Shipside**